THE MAINTENANCE
OF LIFE

Carolina Academic Press
Ethnographic Studies in Medical Anthropology Series
Pamela J. Stewart *and* Andrew Strathern
Series Editors

Curing and Healing
Medical Anthropology in Global Perspective
Andrew Strathern *and* Pamela J. Stewart

Elusive Fragments
Making Power, Propriety and Health in Samoa
Douglass D. Drozdow-St. Christian

Endangered Species
Health, Illness, and Death Among Madagascar's People of the Forest
Janice Harper

The Practice of Concern
Ritual, Well-Being, and Aging in Rural Japan
John W. Traphagan

The Gene and the Genie
Tradition, Medicalization and Genetic Counseling
in a Bedouin Community in Israel
Aviad E. Raz

Social Discord and Bodily Disorders
Healing Among the Yupno of Papua New Guinea
Verena Keck

Indigenous Peoples and Diabetes
Community Empowerment and Wellness
Mariana Leal Ferreira *and* Gretchen Chesley Lang

We Have No Microbes Here
Healing Practices in a Turkish Black Sea Village
Sylvia Wing Önder

Of Orderlies and Men
Hospital Porters Achieving Wellness at Work
Nigel Rapport

The Maintenance of Life
Preventing Social Death through Euthanasia Talk and End-of-Life Care—
Lessons from The Netherlands
Frances Norwood

THE MAINTENANCE OF LIFE

PREVENTING SOCIAL DEATH
THROUGH EUTHANASIA TALK AND
END-OF-LIFE CARE—
LESSONS FROM THE NETHERLANDS

Frances Norwood

CAROLINA ACADEMIC PRESS
Durham, North Carolina

Library of Congress Cataloging-in-Publication Data

Norwood, Frances, 1966-
  The maintenance of life : preventing social death through eu-
thanasia talk and end-of-life care : lessons from the Netherlands /
Frances Norwood.
       p. cm. -- (Ethnographic studies in medical anthropology se-
ries)
  Includes bibliographical references and index.
  ISBN 978-1-59460-518-5 (alk. paper)
  1. Euthanasia--Netherlands. 2. Terminal care--Netherlands. 3.
Medical anthropology. I. Title. II. Series.

R726.N67 2009
179.7--dc22

                                                    2009022910

CAROLINA ACADEMIC PRESS
700 Kent Street
Durham, North Carolina 27701
Telephone (919) 489-7486
Fax (919) 493-5668
www.cap-press.com

Printed in the United States of America

This is dedicated in loving memory to Frances H. Norwood and all the other mothers and fathers, sisters and brothers, wives and husbands who gave us something really special before they died.

Contents

Figures and Tables

Life and the Process of Death: Meanings and Endings

Andrew Strathern and Pamela J. Stewart[1]

Frances Norwood's deeply thoughtful exploration of euthanasia and related practices in the Netherlands induces us to contemplate how death, the final event in any individual life, is, can be, or should be, dealt with in circumstances when curing sickness or indefinitely prolonging that life are not perceived options. The end of life, like the beginning of it, is always potentially difficult, even traumatic, for the network of kin and friends as well as for the dying person. Its meaning must be very different in contexts where cosmological visions imply an afterlife from those in which such visions are attenuated or absent. And attitudes to euthanasia, as well as to suicide, must vary with cosmology also (for an example from the Pacific see Stewart and Strathern 2003). If life is a gift from an omnipotent God, it may be argued that only that God can determine when it should end, and it can thus be expressed in phrases of acceptance such as "It was his/her time", or "an act of God". So, too, with life's beginnings, in conception and parturition. Abortion and euthanasia stand logically in similar spaces of indeterminacy or disapproval, depending on the prevailing cosmology. The Christian doctrinal background in many places, including the Netherlands, would lead to such a presupposition. And in addition to religion the state and its authority over people are likely to be involved. For reasons that must have to do with deeply held predispositions, abortion (under specific circumstances) may be permitted in practice by the state whereas euthanasia is not. At the end of life an adult person has long been enmeshed in the politico-legal structures of the state, their identities and potentialities categorized, filed, and put into place.

Their death, then, may be thought of as belonging more to the state than the termination of life prior to a birth. But, with progressive secularization and rationalization of practices, the state may come to embrace, and at the same time circumscribe practices previously tabooed by custom or religion. The term euthanasia itself implies something that is "good", from its Greek roots, "well-dying" (parallel with "well-being, we might say). The term also carries an echo of the concept of "the good death", defined differently in different culture-historical ways, but sometimes implying a peaceful end, without undue suffering, of a person surrounded by sympathetic kin and friends, who will also give the person, once passed away, a "good funeral".

Issues of terminal care may be involved. When should care become palliative rather than an aggressive attempt to cure a condition? The voluntary choice of a person to move from hospital to home or hospice is a mark of a decision to let life go. Euthanasia, in concept, takes this move one step further, by making death a matter of personal agency rather than a passive acceptance of events that must be considered beyond one's control and allowed to take their course. A decision of a person who feels that their life is effectively at an end simply to die without any artificial assistance at all is sometimes portrayed in works of art, and is not classified as euthanasia, although it is that person's active effort to achieve a good death as they see it. A person may be kept in a nursing home for a long time and remain passively in existence until some minor condition may end their life. They may have willed this or even looked forward to the end, signaling this by an unwillingness to interact much even with kin, or by choosing which kin to interact with and which not as a mark of their continuing agency. When they finally pass away, perhaps in sleep, the event is likely to be described as "a blessing in disguise".

In all or most of these cases the actions of care-givers and visitors are bound up with the idea of compassion. Medicines are administered to alleviate pain or induce sleep. The person's agency and experience become constrained. It is in circumstances like this or when such circumstances are already envisioned or anticipated that discussions about the eventuality of death are likely to reach into people's consciousness. Until then, a patient may be expected to, or may expect to, fight for life, a fight which begins as a fight to get well, to be cured, and may continue as a self-sustaining fight for each succeeding day of existence itself.

Frances Norwood has looked into these issues and processes in both the Netherlands and the U.S.A. Her carefully constructed investigation is also in part framed by her own reflexive subjectivity in relation to the deaths of her own kin, with an increment of empathy resulting from her own experience. The duality of the anthropologist as observer ("subject") and the people she studies as observed ("object") is here definitively transcended. (An even more striking example of this process can be found when an anthropologist discusses and analyzes their own experience with a particular condition, such as Emily Martin (2007) has done in her book on bipolar disorder, in the course of discussing the same topic in a broader fashion.) Norwood explicitly lets us see in her own life some of the concerns that others see and she has studied in theirs, that is, the experience of the deaths of kin or associates. It is the more compelling because of the inevitability and universality of the experiential issues involved.

From her detailed empirical studies in the Netherlands, Norwood brings forward to our attention two surprising results and one informative factor for making comparisons. The first surprising result is that "euthanasia" is often talked about as a possibility which can occupy the attention of a patient and their social network for a period of time without issuing in an actual decision to carry it out or the final implementation of an act of voluntarily ending the life in question. During this time the life of the person can also be reviewed and reflected on, over and above the possible struggle and pain of daily survival, precisely because of the potentiality of setting a date for the death itself. The process can also be shared rather than one that is only introspective. This gives us the second surprising result, that talk about euthanasia may be seen as having a palliative function, even prolonging life while discussion about it goes on, and keeping the patient alive enough to think about what their life has meant and continues to mean and the circumstances in which they would or would not be content to die. Euthanasia talk is therefore as much about life as it is about death.

A further point — and this is the informative factor referred to above — is that the general medical practitioners (*huisarten* in Dutch) in the Netherlands play a close, sympathetic, and mediating role between the state, the patient, and family and kin in the process of euthanasia talk. The role is authorized by the state, and the doctor will eventually play an active part if the patient decides to go through with the procedure of voluntary death. This places a large responsibility on the doctor, which is fulfilled exactly by the house visits, the lengthy discussions, and the whole process of careful deliberative discussion (*overleg* in Dutch) which Norwood remarks is characteristic of Dutch social culture generally. Given the stereotypical patterns of segmental, single-stranded, impersonal, and routinized interaction with primary care physicians in many contexts in the U.S.A., the model of the caring practitioner who makes home visits and gets to know people well seems to be a very valuable one to keep in mind as also potentially beneficial outside of the contexts Norwood is discussing concerning euthanasia.

The reference to euthanasia talk as a kind of palliative care, in which doctor, patient, and social network co-operate reminds one of the functions of hospice care in many places where euthanasia as such would not be legally permitted. From *The Irish Times* Weekend Review section for Saturday, December 13, 2008 (published in The Republic of Ireland) we culled a lead article with the title "Living and dying with dignity". The article foregrounds the breadth of functions of hospices run by the Irish Hospice Foundation, with the aim of offering "more people comfort, friendship and a second home when they need it most" (loc. cit., p. 1). One patient is prominently quoted as saying: "I had been under the illusion that the hospice was a place to die, but it's not. They make it so pleasant and make you feel like somebody cares" (ibid.). The same article reports a first national survey in Ireland conducted in 2004, in which 67% of people wished to die in their homes, without pain, conscious of those around them and with their "loved ones", i.e. kin or friends (ibid.). Yet, it goes on, in practice two thirds of the approximately 30,000 people who die each year in Ireland are in hospitals at the time of death (ibid.).

Here we interpret further the implications of the newspaper article discussed above. Efforts to increase the numbers of hospices and to expand their range of services are clearly designed, we suggest, to close the evident gap between people's ideal wishes and the limitations of what hospitals can do. Hospices are in between hospital and home. They can provide some professional medication, and they can also be more like a home. In a very broad sense, then, they provide both assisted living and assistance with dying. If to die at home is an ideal, for some people, we may note, euthanasia allows this to happen in a planned way. The patient is not whisked away in an ambulance for heroic surgery or medication, but may quietly prepare or be prepared to die.

The same section of *The Irish Times* featured on its back page (p. 16) a brief report, called "the television story of the week", in a documentary film of the "assisted suicide" (loc. cit., p. 16) of a person who was suffering from motor neuron disease. The theme of "dignity" is replayed here in a different context, since the clinic in Switzerland where the event took place is the "Dignitas Clinic" in Switzerland (ibid.). The film was reported to have shown the patient drinking a lethal dose of barbiturates through a straw, falling asleep, and dying within half an hour. The newspaper reporter writes: "He died in peace, in the presence of his wife" and "with a Swiss doctor and with the film crew" whom the dying person "had invited to witness his parting" (p. 16). The piece ends with "I hope he has found the peace he sought", a secular echo of the liturgical *requiescat in pace*, without its original cosmological implications of the dead waiting in peace for the second coming. The search for peace is clearly a theme shared by these two articles at front and back of *The Irish Times* Weekend Review. Dividing them is the question of the avowed and legitimate means of how such peace may be obtained.

Interest in a case like this reported in *The Irish Times* is transnational. We (AJS and PJS) were in Taiwan on research in December of 2008, and we read another account of this case, reported directly from London, which appeared in *The China Post*, a local newspaper there in Taiwan. This report noted that a British television network came under criticism in the U.K. for screening the film. It notes that "this was the first time British television has shown someone committing assisted suicide" (*The China Post*, Thursday December 11th 2008, p. 2). The man whose death was depicted, who was 59 and partly paralyzed from his condition, had been a University Professor, the report says, and had wanted the film made so that people could see how such a death could be comfortable. He gave as his reason for wishing to die that otherwise he would continue to suffer and to inflict suffering on his family (ibid.). Anti-euthanasia activists, however, declared that it was irresponsible to show the film because to do so would be "euthanasia voyeurism" and "would create a false impression of a growing demand for assisted suicide in Britain" (ibid.). It would also strengthen pressures felt by people about imposing on "loved ones [kin], carers or a society that is short of resources", a campaign group called "Care Not Killing" declared (ibid.). Such reports indicate clearly how controversial the subject is; they also show that it is of great and international public interest. To some extent the issue becomes more difficult with the secularization of society, which opens the way to such debate. To some extent, also, it is due to the ability of medicine to keep people alive or artificially alive. One way and another, the question of whether a person can legitimately be the instrument of ending their own life remains a matter of considerable concern in those countries with relatively long life expectancy figures and relatively advanced medical capacities. Dignity does seem to be a central matter in the debates. The Netherlands rule regarding euthanasia is constructed with this matter in focus. The person who, exercising their free will, has decided to end their own life, is in a structural position analogous to that explored by Giorgio Agamben in his book *Homo Sacer* (1998), a person who cannot legitimately be sacrificed but whose killing also cannot necessarily be punished (Agamben 1998: 81); provided it is carried out in a prescribed way, we might add. Suicide or assisted suicide may be regarded as within the zone of taboo; or simply in the zone of the liminal, on the margins of legitimacy. All of these characterizations reflect the complex feelings that surround the topic and relate it to the overall mystery and liminality of the cycle of life and death, intimately related as well as in a sense opposed, often studied by anthropologists in conjunction with ideas about spirits, ghosts, and the "otherworld" that frames the life-span of the person in society. Attitudes toward death are bound to vary enormously according to ideas of this otherworld of spirits. "Gone to a better place" becomes available as a euphemism in a cosmographic world with an image of a "Heaven" in it. In the same religious world the saying "The wages of Sin is death" hints of the opposite of Heaven, Hell. Where such notions are less strong, or absent, focus is likely to be on the circumstances of death itself, whether it is peaceful or troubled and the like. Still, the idea of a journey can be present, wherever the destination is thought to be. Thus, a funeral well attended by kin and friends may be described as having effected "a good send-off" for the dead person.

Since birth and death, as well as other cyclical events, are tied in with kin relations, the roles of kinsfolk are likely to be crucial. The place of such kin in debates about how terminal illness is to be handled and whether a person can die "at home" is always likely to be significant. In nuclear family situations this burden is quite likely to fall on spouses; or on adult children. The extent of the obligations of such care-givers is by the nature of the relationships involved likely to be difficult to measure, since such obligations are open-ended, universal, and at the same time subject to agreements between those involved. At any rate, as with so much of contemporary life which is not conceptualized as belonging to the realm of kinship as such, in practice kin ties and kin networks tend to be involved in decisions about life and death, and it is within the domains of kinship that the cyclicity of life and death is played out.

Dr. Norwood's study explores these and many other matters with great detail and ethnographic insight. Her book contributes deeply both to applied topics in medical anthropology and to a philosophical anthropology of life and death. Indeed she shows that these two topical arenas are closely connected, since basic philosophical ideas and cognitive schemata, expressed in relational or secular terms, create the contexts in which arguments about euthanasia are fought out. Dr. Norwood recommends that the Netherlands approach to these arguments can fruitfully be considered in other contexts, such as those in the U.S.A. Her work makes a most interesting contribution to discussions in Medical Anthropology and we are very pleased to include it within the Medical Anthropology Series of books with Carolina Academic Press.

Cromie Burn Research Unit, University of Pittsburgh
February 2009
PJS and AJS

Note

(1) Prof. Pamela J. Stewart (Strathern) and Prof. Andrew Strathern are a husband and wife research team in the Department of Anthropology, University of Pittsburgh, and are, respectively, Visiting Research Fellow and Visiting Professor, Department of Anthropology, University of Durham, England. They are also Research Associates in the Research Institute of Irish and Scottish Studies, University of Aberdeen, Scotland, and have been Visiting Research Fellows at the Institute of Ethnology, Academia Sinica, Taipei, Taiwan during parts of 2002, 2003, 2004, 2005, 2006, 2007, and 2008. They have published over 35 books and over 175 articles on their research in the Pacific, Asia (mainly Taiwan), and Europe (primarily Scotland and Ireland). Their most recent co-authored books include *Witchcraft, Sorcery, Rumors, and Gossip* (Cambridge Uni-

versity Press, 2004); and *Self and Group: Kinship in Action* (in preparation with Prentice Hall). Their recent co-edited books include *Exchange and Sacrifice* (Carolina Academic Press, 2008) and *Religious and Ritual Change: Cosmologies and Histories*(Carolina Academic Press, 2009).

Their most recent research is on the topics of Cosmological Landscapes, Religious Conversion, Ritual Studies, and Political Peace-making.

References

Agamben, Giorgio (1998) *Homo Sacer.* Stanford, CA: Stanford University Press.

Martin Emily (2007) *Bipolar Expeditions. Mania and Depression in American Culture.* Princeton, N.J.: Princeton University Press.

Stewart, Pamela J. and Andrew Strathern (2003). The Ultimate Protest Statement: Suicide as a means of defining self-worth among the Duna of the Southern Highlands Province, PNG. *Journal of Ritual Studies* 17.1: 79-88.

Preface

This is a book about how people die today. When I mention to people I meet that I study death and dying, I invariably get one of two responses. Sometimes the person opens up with a heartfelt story of the death of a loved one or the person shys away from the topic with a comment like, "Isn't that depressing?" and nonverbal cues that tell me that they really don't want to know the answer to the question. The answer is yes, death is depressing, but there is also something beautiful and life-affirming about witnessing the passing of a human life. Studying with people who were dying and with people who cared for them taught me something about death, and about life. Death is hard and by witnessing it so intimately, I came to a new understanding of how valuable life is and I learned a little bit more about myself and what I want from life.

This book is about the day-to-day experience of death in a culture that has experimented with some new ways of supporting modern death. This book is for anyone interested in learning more about death in another culture in order to gain some insight into life and death where you live. This book is written for persons who are dying and for the family members who care for them. It is for healthcare professionals, bioethicists, policymakers, anthropologists and other social scientists interested in learning how to make a better way at the end of life.

This book is also intended for those on both sides of the euthanasia and assisted suicide debates. Most chapters begin with an extended excerpt of someone's experience, highlighted by italics in the text. Based on in-depth interviews and observations with patients, family members, and healthcare practitioners, these excerpts provide readers, who both support and oppose assisted dying policies, information about how assisted dying occurs on a day-to-day basis. They include direct quotes from taped interviews with participants (marked in the text by quotations) and paraphrased quotes and observations gained from fieldnotes taken during or immediately following an event and often double-checked by interviews with participants following an event. While individual names have been changed, the stories—the events, the people, and the locations—are real.

Acknowledgments

First and foremost, I would like to thank Anne Mei The and Gerrit van der Wal at the Department of Social Medicine, Free University in Amsterdam and my Dutch advisory committee—Gerrit van der Wal, Anne Mei The, Dick Willems, and Sjaak van der Geest—without whose support I could not have been able to undertake this ethnography. I would like to thank Sharon Kaufman for being such an inspiring mentor and my U.S. dissertation committee for all their support—Sharon Kaufman, Lawrence Cohen, Nelleke Van Deusen-Scholl and Anne-Mei The. Thank you to all my study participants (most of whom must remain nameless) and colleagues who kindly offered comments on chapter drafts—Clive Seale, Chris Ganchoff, Renée Beard, John Griffiths, Peggy Battin, Gerrit Kimsma, Albert Klijn, and Derek Humphry. Thank you to series editors Andrew Strathern and Pamela Stewart for feedback that helped make this book much better than it would have been. Thank you to Kelly Miller, Beth Hall and the staff at Carolina Academic Press for all their help in making this a better manuscript.

Thank you to my mother for inspiring me to seek and to my father for inspiring me to study and learn. Thank you to the *huisartsen* who bravely offered to have an American anthropologist in tow. Finally, thank you to all the families who participated in this study who opened their homes and their lives to me when they had such precious little time left together. This project has received funding through grants from the University of California-San Francisco, University of California-Berkeley, the American Association for Netherlandic Studies, and the Netherland-America Foundation. Any mistakes in this text are my own.

Chapters 1 and 2 include excerpts of an article reprinted by permission from Taylor & Francis Ltd (Norwood, Frances 2007 Nothing More To Do: Euthanasia, General Practice, and End-of-Life Discourse in The Netherlands." *Medical Anthropology* 26(2):139–174). Chapter 4 is based on an article reprinted by permission from the editor of *Medische Antropologie* (Norwood, Frances 2006 A Hero and a Criminal: Dutch Huisartsen and the Making of Good Death Through Euthanasia Talk in The Netherlands. *Medische Antropologie* 18(2):329–347).

THE MAINTENANCE
OF LIFE

CHAPTER 1

THAT'S NOT MY WIFE

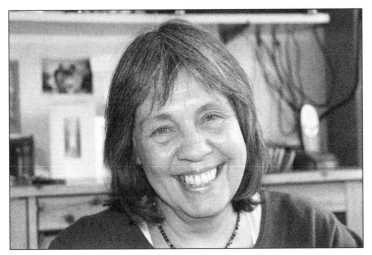

Photo credit: Nicole Marshall

To anyone who has ever lived in another country for an extended period of time, you will recall the culture shock of experiencing a different way of life. I remember one such shock very distinctly. I was standing in the living room of one of those small, quaint Dutch houses and the man of the house was showing me pictures of his family. His wife was ill with terminal cancer and had come home from the hospital to die among family. He turned to his wife lying sick in the bed and he said to me, "That's not my wife. My wife, she's here," and he held up a framed photograph of her in his hand.

To get to his house I rode my bicycle from Amsterdam to what quickly transforms into Dutch countryside, complete with stretches of green pastures, the smell of cows, the ever-present canal and the occasional windmill. I was in a small country on the edge of Europe, called The Netherlands. Often I notice in the U.S. when I mention having lived in The Netherlands, a surprising number of people have difficulty placing the country. "Is that where they speak Danish?" they often ask. Part of the confusion I think can be blamed on the English translation of their name. In the Dutch language, the country is *Nederland,* the language is *Nederlands* and the people are *Nederlanders,* but in English, the language and the people are "Dutch," and the country is alternately referred to as The Netherlands, the Lowlands, or Holland.[1]

I think, however, it is more than just a name that confuses people. Situated between Germany, Belgium and the North Sea, The Netherlands is a country whose tourist image teeters between an idyllic and bucolic past made up of tulips, windmills, canals and wooden clogs and a progressive and sometimes harsh modernity that often centers around its best known city, Amsterdam, and its somewhat radical social policies regulating access to prostitution, soft drugs, homosexual marriage and euthanasia. Amsterdam is a beautiful old city that is dominated by canals, bicycles and the tall, thin houses and architecture of the 17th century, their "Golden Age." This merges, however, with some very modern alterations. Just take a walk up the Damrak from Central Station and you can see the past clashing with the present. The narrow streets are filled with people, bicycles, cars and trams, the smell of food and the bustle of movement cut only by the unusual scent of hash coming from a number of "brown" cafes, called coffee shops. In the Leidseplein, Burger King is nestled next to the Bull Dog, one of the original brown cafes where you can buy and smoke soft drugs such as hash and marijuana in what, ironically, was an old police station. Turn left and you make your way through the Red Light District, where you will pass the most pic-

---

1. The name "Holland," which is used sometimes by Dutch people and often by outsiders is not an accurate name for the country and is even offensive to some Dutch residents. "Holland" technically refers to only two of seven provinces in The Netherlands (North and South Holland), which makes up many, but not all, of the key Dutch cities and does not include the majority of the Dutch countryside.

turesque canals, old churches and 17th century row houses, yet be surrounded by sex shops, brown cafes and bars, hawkers advertising live sex shows, and the signature neon windows of the Red Light District where prostitutes put themselves on display for potential customers and the many tourists who flock there to see what is typically left out of the public eye in their own countries.

No question, The Netherlands is a unique country and Amsterdam a unique place. But the Dutch share something with Americans and others from around the world that is important. They, like us, die and before they die they too struggle to maintain life, family, and identity—to maintain connection with the social fabric that makes up a distinctly Dutch society. I was shocked that a man would say at the foot of his own wife's bed that she was not his wife, but when he pointed to the photo from the past he asked me to understand something that impacts all of us.

When people die suddenly or unexpectedly, the family is left to deal with the loss of their loved one. Through mourning rituals, funerals, and a myriad of other organized and informal social supports, family members walk through their loss. With advances in medicine, people are living longer, but that often means that they are living longer with chronic conditions, physical and social limitations and losses. Physician and end-of-life researcher Joanne Lynn compares U.S. deaths in 1900 with deaths in 2000 to demonstrate how much death has changed. The average life expectancy in 1900 was 47 and most people at that time died at home from infections or accidents, experiencing at most hours or weeks of decline before death. Compare that to figures from today and you find that life expectancy and living with chronic illness have both increased dramatically. Today, life expectancy in the U.S. averages around 75 years and people are most likely to die in the hospital, funded in part by Medicare, with an average of two years of chronic conditions and decline (Lynn 2004:1–10).

What happens when living and dying become something that is drawn out? Often both those who are ill and their close friends and family members deal with a series of losses. These losses do not follow any one set trajectory, but there are patterns in the types of decline and the losses that generally occur. Lynn characterizes three types of dying trajectories that occur as a result of chronic illness today. There is the short period of decline that often occurs with some types of cancer, severe stroke and certain AIDS cases. There is the long-term decline that occurs with intermittent periods of serious decline and partial recovery that is typical of persons with organ system failure, such as congestive heart failure, lung disease or kidney failure. And then there is the prolonged decline that occurs most often with general frailty or dementia, such as Alzheimer's (Lynn 2004:44–50).

Individuals who are sick or dying may lose the ability to work, to read, to bathe themselves, to go to the bathroom on their own, to walk, to talk, to eat. Each individual may experience differences in the severity and duration of these losses. Some may maintain the ability to eat and do self-care up until the last week; some may live for years in a near vegetative state relying on respirators and artificial feeding. What all of these losses have in common is that they are based in social activities—activities that, even though they are necessary for biological life, typically impact one's ability to participate in their social environment. These are the kinds of losses that lead up to a man saying that a photograph is a better representation of his wife, than the woman lying in the bed herself.

Social Death

There is a term for what the man with the photograph is describing: that term is *social death*. The origin of the term social death is a little unclear. It was first attributed to sociologist Erving Goffman by one of his students as an example of the "predeath treatment" of mental patients found in mental institutions of that era.[2] In *Asylums* (1961), Goffman describes what happens to pa-

---

2. While I cannot find direct reference of the term in Goffman's work, I see that Goffman was a supervisor at the University of California-Berke-

tients newly admitted to a mental institution, observing that patients start with "relationships and rights," but end up through the course of their in-patient treatment with "hardly any of either" (Goffman 1961:133).

In 1965, sociologists Barney Glaser and Anselm Strauss (1965) used the term to describe a practice whereby hospital patients are informally evaluated by staff as deserving or undeserving of care. Glaser and Strauss suggest that patients had to demonstrate certain social attributes or risk a type of social death, or shunning, by staff. Goffman's student David Sudnow used the term in a slightly different way in his study of hospital death. In *Passing On* (1967), Sudnow found evidence of a kind of social death, which he defines as the point prior to biological or clinical death at which a patient is essentially treated as a corpse; the point at which "socially relevant attributes of the patient begin permanently to cease to be operative as conditions for treating him, and when he is, essentially, regarded as already dead" (Sudnow 1967:74). One chilling example Sudnow gives is a nurse who spent two to three minutes attempting to close the eyes of a dying patient. When questioned about what she was doing, she explained that it was easier to achieve a complete closure of the eyelids if she closed the eyes of patients before death and before rigor mortis set in (Sudnow 1967:74).

For the purposes of my study, social death cannot be attributed to a single point in time, nor attributed to a strict set of behaviors. It is probably best described as a series of losses—loss of identity and loss of the ability to participate in social activities and relationships that eventually culminates in a perceived disconnection from social life. For the man whose wife was in the photograph, a social death had occurred. Yet even that is not absolute. He may again see glimpses of the wife he knew, she may awaken to share a

---

ley for Sudnow's dissertation research to study death in the hospital and it is possible that David Sudnow may be referring to a personal communication when he attributes to Goffman the origination of the term, *social death* (Sudnow 1967:v, 72).

few moments of connection with her loved ones, and every person in her life, including she herself, may have a different and shifting perceptions of what constitutes social death.

What is clear is that the landscape of death and dying has changed. Today, death most often does not happen in an instant, it is more typically a long process of life mixed in with decline and social losses that eventually (sometimes many years after an initial onset of terminal or serious illness) culminates in some combination of social and biological death. When death and dying changes, then so too must our practices at the end of life change. British sociologist Clive Seale (1998) talks about changes that have occurred in many places around the world in response to the prolongation of life and the shifting experience of death. Building on the work of Thomas Scheff (1990), Seale suggests that maintenance of social bonds is a basic human urge. According to Seale, late modernity has seen the rise of at least two strategies for maintaining social bonds. The first strategy is a kind of therapeutic discourse, where the aware dying person is able to transform social losses that occur at the end of life into a meaningful script and through this process the person is able to maintain a level of agency and social connection through the dying process. Seale explains,

> Here, people with terminal disease have the opportunity to construct themselves as inner adventurers, transforming the experience of dying into an opportunity for personal growth and an affirmation of caring bonds, gaining entry to temporary liminal communities such as those constructed in hospice care, aided by professional members of the caring team (Seale 1998:7).

According to Seale, a second strategy for maintaining social bonds today is by euthanasia or assisted dying, where patients make the decision to alter the exact time of biological death to have it coincide more closely with social death (Seale 1998:7–8). In other words, when the woman in the bed is no longer a valid representation of her social being as perceived by those around her (herself included), then euthanasia or assistance in dying can be used to literally relocate death of the body to coincide with the point in time where her sociality ends.

A Study of Dutch End of Life

In the summer of 1999, with not much more than the names of two Dutch colleagues and a handful of Dutch language classes under my belt, I traveled to The Netherlands to test Seale's ideas about social death and to see if I could find out more about death and dying in the country that is known for its end-of-life policy. The Netherlands is the country with the longest standing legal practice of euthanasia and assisted suicide, legalizing these practices by court decision in 1984 and by law in 2002. Today, euthanasia (killing a person at that person's explicit request typically for reasons of incurable illness) is legally practiced in The Netherlands (since 1984), Belgium (since 2002), and, most recently, Luxembourg (since 2009). Assisted suicide (providing a person with the means to kill themselves typically for reasons of incurable illness)[3] is legally practiced in The Netherlands (since 1984), Belgium (since 2002), Luxembourg (since 2009), Switzerland (since 1937) and in the state of Oregon in the United States (since 1997). In 2008, voters in the state of Washington passed Initiative 1000, legalizing physician-assisted suicide in that state as well. The Netherlands is not the first country in the modern era to legalize euthanasia by law (Australia legalized euthanasia for a brief period in 1995), but it is the first

---

3. Every country defines euthanasia, assisted suicide, and other medical behavior at the end of life differently. These terms and definitions for euthanasia and assisted suicide are how these practices are talked about and defined by current Dutch policy. Throughout this text I may use the term "euthanasia" to include euthanasia and assisted suicide in reference to the Dutch practice as outlined in Dutch law. In reference to the U.S. practice, I will use the term "physician-assisted dying (PAD)" or assisted dying to best match terminology used in the Oregon law. For more on varying definitions for these and other end of life practices, see Chapter 3.

country to legally practice euthanasia and, with over 20 years of legal practice, it is the country most often held as the model for or against euthanasia policies in other countries (Goldstein 2008; Heide, et al. 2003; SCBI 2002; Scherer and Simon 1999).[4]

As a lone American researcher in Amsterdam, I was frequently asked why I would want to do such a study. There were several reasons. As a graduate student of anthropology studying to get my PhD at the University of California-San Francisco and Berkeley, this was my chance to be initiated in the experience of my forefathers (and mothers!), to move to a new land and learn the ways, language and customs of a new place and people. I had always wanted to return to The Netherlands. I had been there twice before, once briefly on a month long backpack trip across Europe that seemed to allow only enough time to carry my own culture through the many cities and towns we visited. The second time, I went as a graduate assistant where I assisted in a summer field school program to teach American college students about the criminal justice system in England and The Netherlands. I remember very well what initially struck me about the Dutch people. After touring several dark and dismal prisons in England, we arrived in The Netherlands. While there were Dutch prisons that were also depressing, the Dutch system seemed to have a slightly different take on criminality and what constitutes personhood. I remember one visit to a Dutch prison in particular. The prison guard took us on a tour of the cell blocks. For the first time

---

4. There is a lot of play between law and practice. For example, euthanasia was legalized by court ruling in Colombia in 1997 and in Germany assisted suicide has been technically legal since 1751. In both countries, however, euthanasia and assisted suicide as I have defined these terms are rarely ever practiced or occur only in private due to strong societal or religious taboos. Conversely, in some of the Scandinavian countries, there are no laws allowing assisted suicide, yet it is a practice known to occur behind closed doors and, like in many countries, the sanctions against someone accused tend not to be severe. For this reason, I am choosing to use the term, *legally practiced*, to denote both legal precedence and transparency of practice (Scherer and Simon 1999).

in our tour of prisons, I watched as the guard knocked on a prisoner's door and asked if we could come in. The prisoner answered the door just as if it were his own house, graciously letting us peep inside the small space. That very simple gesture by the guard communicated a kind of respect for the man in the cell that I began to see echoed in our visits in other Dutch prisons, courts, work release programs, and community policing in the Red Light District of Amsterdam. The Netherlands seemed to be a vastly different place than the U.S., where prisoners are afforded some respect and privacy; where issues of criminality regarding euthanasia, prostitution and use of soft drugs are redefined; and where Dutch citizens are ensured access to healthcare, regardless of their ability to pay. What lessons could we learn from these striking societal differences?

Beginning in 1999, I returned to The Netherlands to take the first in a series of immersion Dutch language courses and to explore possibilities for research. Using my two contacts, I began to meet many of the researchers who study euthanasia. Through anthropologist Sjaak van der Geest, I met medical anthropologist Anne Mei The, one of only two researchers who had conducted ethnographic (observation-based) research on euthanasia. The [pronounced "teh"] introduced me to Gerrit van der Wal, chair of the Department of Social Medicine at the Free University of Amsterdam and one of the head researchers of the on-going nationwide (and now international) quantitative study of the prevalence and incidence of euthanasia and other medical behaviors at the end of life. I do not know if it was my determination to speak Dutch during these meetings (no matter how inadequate my skills initially were) or my determination in general, but both The and van der Wal agreed to support my research and before summer's end, we had assembled a team of physicians and researchers to discuss the possibilities of my doing the next ethnographic study of euthanasia.

What was clear was that an observation-based study was sorely needed. Most of the research on euthanasia and assisted suicide from around the world tends to be based on quantitative (survey) research or interview research conducted predominantly with physicians (Emanuel, et al. 2000; Ganzini 2004; Hendin 1997; Pearlman and Starks 2004; Sprung, et al. 2006; van der Heide, et al. 2007; Ward and Tate 1994). These kinds of studies can tell you generally how many cases of euthanasia exist or what opinions physicians share about end-of-life practices, but cannot reveal how euthanasia actually occurs on a daily basis or describe the experience that patients and families share. Since the first two ethnographic studies of euthanasia were based in the hospital (Pool 1996; The 1997),[5] mine would be based in the home and nursing home (*verzorgingshuis*) where the majority of euthanasia deaths occur via the general practitioner, or *huisarts*. In 2001, 77 percent of all euthanasia and 87 percent of all assisted suicide deaths were handled by *huisartsen* (Wal, et al. 2003:46). I also included in my sample one *verpleegarts* who worked in a combination nursing home (*verzorgingshuis*) and 24-hour acute nursing home (*verpleeghuis*). After more Dutch language lessons, a month-long pilot study in Amsterdam to test the feasibility of a home-based study, and after securing funding and IRB approval both at my university and (as an added safety measure) at the Free University in Amsterdam, I was ready to begin.[6]

---

5. South African anthropologist Robert Pool (1996)and Dutch medical anthropologist Anne Mei The (1997) wrote the first two, full length, observation-based ethnographies of euthanasia in modern times. Pool's ethnography focuses on the experience of the physician and The's focuses on the experience of the nurse. Both were conducted in Dutch hospitals and both were originally available only in the Dutch language. Pool has since written another version of his original ethnography, which is now available in the English language (2000).

6. Being able to speak and understand the Dutch language was critical to my study. Even though the Dutch people are known for being fluent in English and often several other languages, prior experience working with end-of-life patients showed me that when a person is very sick, it often becomes difficult to speak a second language. Also, I really wanted to capture the Dutch experience in their own words and since much of my time would be spent observing physicians and patients together, I did not want to regularly interrupt those interactions for translation. Prior to my study, I completed three years of Dutch language study, including three intensive language courses in The Netherlands and one-on-one in-

In the summer of 2000, I moved to Amsterdam to start what would become a 15-month ethnographic study of euthanasia, general practice, and home-based death in The Netherlands. From 1999 to 2001, I conducted observations and interviews with 15 physicians—14 general practitioners (*huisartsen*), one acute care nursing home physician (*verpleegarts*) and approximately 650 of their general population patients. I also conducted intensive case study research with 10 of the 14 *huisartsen* and 25 of their end-of-life patients (14 with euthanasia requests and 11 without). Case study participants were tracked more intensively and the work included multiple observations, interviews (taped and not taped) and/or survey research with patients, families, physicians, and home care employees over the course of the person's lifetime or until the completion of the study year.

The literal translation of the word, *huisarts,* is "physician of the house or home" and that is not far from the truth. Dutch *huisartsen,* I found, are quite different from their American counterparts. In spite of a push in many advanced medical cultures towards a technology- and efficiency-driven system of medical care, Dutch *huisartsen* typically conduct a number of house calls daily (according to my research, an average 7 out of 28 daily patient visits are conducted in the home or nursing home). In their interactions with patients and families, *huisartsen* have a tendency to favor a more holistic, discussion-based practice. It is not that they do not have access to the latest technologies and treatments, they do; rather it is that the healthcare system and cultural norms currently support a more home- and talk-centered style of general practice. So to distinguish Dutch *huisartsen* from their American counterparts, you will see me use the Dutch term, *huisarts* (pl. *huisartsen*) throughout this text to remind readers that general practice in your home country may not be the same as general practice in The Netherlands.

---

struction with a native speaker. During my stay in The Netherlands, I continued my language study, which turned out to be a good way to make friends and to further hone my language skills. Nearly all interviews and observations were conducted in the Dutch language.

In addition to research with *huisartsen,* patients and families, I conducted interviews with more than 35 researchers, physicians, and advocates on both sides of the euthanasia debate to better understand the Dutch health care system and the cultural context in which euthanasia and end-of-life practices occur (see Appendix A). The Dutch have a system of healthcare based in social medicine, in which healthcare services are available on a sliding scale fee or free-of-charge to those who cannot afford it. During my study, the Dutch insurance system consisted of public and private sector funding streams that gave coverage to almost 100 percent of the population. Anyone below a certain salary (€31,750 gross per year in 2003) was covered by *Ziekenfonds,* the government subsidized, but privately managed insurance system, which covered approximately two-thirds of the population. The Dutch system includes the AWBZ (*Algemene Wet Bijzondere Ziektekosten,* or the General Law for Extraordinary Medical Costs), which is available to anyone to cover the cost of nursing home care, home care and medical equipment. Dutch people also have access to *Thuiszorg,*[7] the national homecare service, which provides nursing and personal care services in the home up to four times per day, including overnight respite. While waitlists for homecare and specialty services are common, those who are dying typically receive the services they request because they are moved up on waitlists as they demonstrate higher need.

On January 1, 2006, the Dutch passed healthcare reform, changing to a single, compulsory system of national health care insurance for all. It is a new system of 'managed competition,' which keeps general practitioners as the gatekeepers, but allows consumers freedom to change their insurer and insurance plan. The new payment system for general practitioners includes annual capitation

---

7. *Thuiszorg* is also available on a sliding scale fee or free-of-charge to those who need it. Typically, however, there is a waitlist for homecare services. There are reasons that patients will be moved up the waitlist, including demonstrated need at the end of life. Approximately half of my case study sample of patients who chose to die at home were receiving *Thuiszorg* services (Norwood 2005:131).

payments per patient and a fee per consult (both available under the former system), plus reimbursement for costs related to type of service rendered, staff employed, and quality and efficiency indicators (Griffiths, et al. 2008:15–23; Grol 2006; Weel 2004).

To understand the larger healthcare system and the context of home-based case, I conducted observation and interviews with *Thuiszorg* (the national Dutch home care), *Hospice Kuria* (the Amsterdam hospice facility), and in independent living facilities (*aanleunwoning*), nursing homes (*verzorgingscentra*), elder care homes (*bejaardenhuizen*) and acute care facilities (*verpleeghuizen*) where patients receive 24-hour acute care. The bulk of my research activities, however, focused on intensive observation and interviews with 10 *huisartsen* (half in the city of Amsterdam and half in a cluster of small towns outside of Amsterdam) and 25 of their end-of-life patients and their families, 14 with euthanasia requests and 11 without.

A typical research day was spent conducting interviews in the morning and observation on house calls with *huisartsen* in the afternoon. Dutch general practice is generally divided into two parts: morning and afternoon. Morning generally consisted of back-to-back office visits, averaging approximately 12½ minutes each. The bulk of the office visits were usually done in the morning, broken up by a coffee break at 10:15, and completed occasionally by one or a handful of house calls, or home visits. *Huisartsen* in the city generally biked to their house calls. Due to greater distances, their town counterparts all conducted house calls by car. Afternoons were typically slower (fewer patients) and office visits generally lasted longer (more complex and psychosocial problems are intentionally scheduled for the afternoon). Afternoons might include an hour of phone consultations (when patients can call in to talk to the *huisarts* personally) and typically include the bulk of the home visits.

Initially, I conducted participant observation with *huisartsen* throughout the day as they saw patients in their office and on house calls. Later, I focused more on observation during house calls to maximize the time spent with patients who were terminal or dying. Through periodic observation and telephone updates throughout the study year with *huisartsen*, I met their end-of-life patients (persons who were terminal, dying or had an active request for euthanasia). Sometimes patients were no longer able to communicate and in that case a family member might agree to participate. Once a patient and their family were brought into the study, I continued observation on house calls with the *huisarts* and on my own I would return for interviews with patients, families, and sometimes other healthcare professionals, such as *Thuiszorg* homecare employees who were frequently in the home. For some who died soon after we met, this meant only a few visits or interviews; for others who lived longer, this meant periodic visits throughout the duration of the study. Observation notes were taken either during the visit or in between each patient visit and then handwritten notes were expanded in electronic form within 72 hours of an event. Formal interviews were taped and later transcribed by a native Dutch speaker. All translations are my own.

Several different methods were used to ensure data quality. Triangulation of sources was used to check the validity and reliability of data collected. For example, each observation event included a reliability check via a short interview with the *huisarts* to confirm the accuracy and consistency of researcher observations. For the 25 intensive case studies, multiple data sources were used, including multiple observations and interviews with multiple participants. In addition, each *huisarts* completed an exit interview at the conclusion of each case study and a case study survey at the conclusion of the study year to verify the accuracy of data collected.

Throughout the research, I relied on a team of expert advisors in The Netherlands and in the U.S. My Dutch Advisory Committee[8] assisted in the development of study methodology prior to beginning the study and met periodically throughout the study to

---

8. My Dutch advisory committee included Anne Mei The, PhD, author of *Vanavond Om 8 Uur* [*This Evening at 8*], one of two ethnographies on Dutch euthanasia; Gerrit van der Wal, MD, co-author of the nationwide study on the incidence and prevalence of euthanasia in The Netherlands and former chair of the Department of Social Medicine at the Free University in Amsterdam; Dick Willems, MD, *huisarts* and bioethicist; and

review and discuss common and outlier cases, to discuss and refine data collection activities, and to review preliminary study findings. My U.S. dissertation committee[9] assisted in the conceptualization of the research prior to and following data collection activities and provided feedback during data collection in response to analysis memos submitted via electronic mail. Surviving case study participants were given drafts of early publications and were asked to offer corrections and make comments, confirming the accuracy of individual case study details. Finally, study findings were presented to researchers, physicians and other social scientists in both The Netherlands and the U.S. via conference papers (Norwood 2001a; Norwood 2001b; Norwood 2001c; Norwood 2006c) and via publications (Norwood 2006b; Norwood 2007). Comments received from experts from around the world suggest that although this is a small, qualitative sample from the greater Amsterdam region, findings may be valid to a larger geographic area (Griffiths et al. 2008:185–6; Kimsma and Leeuwen 2007; Weyers 2006). Overall findings should be considered suggestive, but not necessarily conclusive of common medical behaviors at the end of Dutch life.

The bulk of this ethnography relies on qualitative research completed in The Netherlands. Comparisons with the American experience rely on secondary sources, a 12-month qualitative study with chaplains working in a university teaching hospital (Norwood 2006a), 14 years experience conducting research on long term care for persons with disabilities (Harrington, et al. 2001; Norwood 1996), and personal experience gained from volunteering with hospice in the U.S. and as a family member researching care options for my parents.

Sjaak van der Geest, PhD, medical anthropologist and chair of the Medical Anthropology Unit at the University of Amsterdam.

9. My dissertation committee included Sharon Kaufman, PhD, medical anthropologist at the University of California-San Francisco and author of *And a Time to Die,* an ethnography of hospital death; Lawrence Cohen, PhD, medical anthropologist at the University of California-Berkeley; Nelleke Van Deusen-Scholl, PhD, Dutch linguist at the University of Pennsylvania; and Anne Met The, PhD, medical anthropologist formerly with the Free University in Amsterdam.

The Book

After 15 months in The Netherlands, what I found was not what I expected. *First my study revealed that euthanasia in practice is predominantly a discussion that only rarely culminates in a euthanasia death. In practice, it is predominantly a discourse grounded in cultural and historical norms that shape how Dutch people have come to think, feel and act at the end of life.* What are Dutch people talking about when they talk about euthanasia? Part I of this book puts euthanasia talk and euthanasia death into theoretical, cultural and historical perspectives. Using extended quotations from observation notes and interviews, I attempt to give readers on both sides of the debate for and against euthanasia, data they can use to make up their own mind. My analysis begins in Chapter 2 where I describe euthanasia talk and illuminate this talk as evidence of a response to social death. Part I starts with the story of euthanasia that tends to receive the most attention in the media; it is the story of one woman's euthanasia death. In Chapter 2, I compare this with a story that is more typical of the Dutch experience with euthanasia: the story of one woman's experience as she explores euthanasia as an end-of-life option. Using these examples in the context of data from the entire study sample, I will begin the process of breaking down just what the Dutch do when they participate in euthanasia talk and euthanasia death. Chapter 2 gives the reader an introduction to the framework of euthanasia talk as a discourse — what it consists of, who participates, and how — and introduces the concept of 'discourse' taken from Michel Foucault in *The Archaeology of Knowledge* (1972) and in two of his later works (1978; 1991). According to Foucault, discourses are scripts that emerge in societies. They are cultural forms that shape the way we think, feel and act. They limit what can be spoken, what is constituted as taboo, what is held in collective conscience, what is reconstituted from the past, and who in society has access. Using Foucault's framework of discourse as a way to look at end-of-life practices and Seale's ideas about responses to social death

(1998), I will offer clues to what discussions and practices occur at the end of Dutch life and why.

Practices are embedded in culture and history, so to understand Dutch euthanasia, the cultural and historical processes and events that led up to its current form are of particular analytical significance. In Chapter 3, we will examine euthanasia as it has existed in various forms through culture and history. Taking a closer look through history reveals two very interesting points. First, euthanasia has long been associated with suicide, often categorized as one of the more acceptable forms of suicide, for reasons of altruism, honor, sickness or old age. Throughout history and across cultures, suicide has often been viewed as taboo, thus the link between suicide and euthanasia carries some real consequences. Secondly, it is interesting that euthanasia and other medical behaviors at the end of life are only recently coming under regulation. Think of it, euthanasia is a practice that has existed at least as far back as our written and oral records indicate (Lam 1997). It is also a practice that is known to occur today behind closed doors in countries where it is not yet fully regulated, including across the U.S. (Emanuel 1994; Emanuel, et al. 2000; Humphry 1978; Lam 1997; Magnusson 2004; Rollin 1987; Shavelson 1995). Chapter 3 will explore why euthanasia and assisted suicide is only recently coming under the scrutiny of medicine and law.

Modern day euthanasia and other medical behaviors at the end of life are not just practices rooted in history, they are practices rooted in culture. Attempts to criticize Dutch policies on the end-of-life or to transfer these policies to other countries cannot proceed without some understanding of the impact of culture. What is culture? Increasingly anthropologists are shying away from the term, because increasingly we see the concept of culture limited by its use as a noun. Many anthropologists now believe that to label a group of people or a geographic place as one unified and bound 'culture' is no longer a useful tool for understanding why people do the things they do. Culture, per se, does not exist as something that can be defined by who is a member or by borders that delineate race, class, nation, or proximity (Behar and Gordon 1995; Clifford and Marcus 1986). Dutch culture and American culture, in essence, do not exist.

A different way to look at culture is to focus not on a set of characteristics shared by a set group of people, but on some of the common processes (development and transference of behaviors, knowledge, and attitudes) exhibited by persons who share defining characteristics, events, or location. Culture is something that is shared, but not always equally. It is fragmentary and both impacts and is impacted by people who share something—be it race, ethnicity, gender, ancestry, geography, nationhood (the list could go on). Culture shapes commonly held understandings of how things are and how things should be, and these are understandings that are passed down through generations, constantly being re-interpreted, re-worked, and re-defined.

Culture is most visible when you visit a new place. Many Dutch people share a favored pastime with foreigners like myself; they love to discuss with new arrivals what is and is not 'typically Dutch.' While I believe that no one characteristic can be attributed to all Dutch people or even most of the people in the greater Amsterdam region (the site of my study), I will argue in this book that there are understandings that are typical. In Chapter 3, I will introduce the reader to several 'typically Dutch' cultural processes that are impacting euthanasia and Dutch end of life. There is the Dutch tendency towards *overleg* (consultation) and the very unique *huisarts*-patient relationship, which is based in dialogue. *Overleg* is a process for decision-making that is used broadly in The Netherlands in which each participant has an equal voice and a decision is made, usually diluted by compromise and majority rule. Chapter 3 explores some of the consequences of end-of-life practices based in dialogue and compromise.

There is also a Dutch emphasis on order and control. The Netherlands has a long history of controlling nature. As much as one-third of the country now exists as land because the Dutch have reclaimed it from beneath the sea by a massive system of dykes, pumps, and polders. Could the Dutch willingness to control water (nature) be linked to their willingness to control death (nature) by euthanasia policy? And if euthanasia talk and euthanasia death are not the same thing, then just what are the Dutch making orderly through these euthanasia practices? Finally, I found that faith seemed to be impacting Dutch end-of-life, but not in the way I expected. In the U.S., our debates around euthanasia tend to be debates often framed in moral and religious terms. In The Netherlands, where they have spent the last 30 years debating euthanasia that is no longer how the majority of the debate is framed. The Dutch focus is on working out the details of legal practice and during my stay in The Netherlands much of the debate was on how to ensure that physicians report euthanasia properly and where the borders of legal practice should lie.

What happened to the moral debate in The Netherlands and what role does faith or religion now play in a country where euthanasia is largely accepted? My research suggests that secularization has left a space that may have been replaced by a faith in society to take care of its own. Of all the EU countries, The Netherlands has, since the 1970s, experienced one of the highest rates of secularization. What was once a stronghold for Catholicism and later Calvinism has changed. In Chapter 3, I will talk about how this vacuum left by the rather abrupt move away from the Catholic and Protestant establishments may have provided the Dutch with an opportunity to replace faith in God with faith in society and the processes that society have created to manage Dutch life.

My second major finding exposes an interesting irony, that euthanasia talk in many ways serves a palliative function, prolonging life and staving off social death by providing participants with a venue for processing meaning, giving voice to suffering, and reaffirming social bonds and self-identity at the end of Dutch life. In talking euthanasia, dying individuals are provided with the social resources they need to remain connected through the difficult course of a final illness. This, I argue, is one reason why so many Dutch people talk about euthanasia, but then choose not to go through with it.

In Part II, I focus on the Dutch experience with euthanasia and examine euthanasia talk as a means for social affirmation and bonding via the roles that participants assume and anticipate in end-of-life discussions. Chapter 4 focuses on the *huisarts* and the distinct role that they play at the end of Dutch life. This chapter begins with the reflections of one *huisarts* as he explores what it means to perform euthanasia. We know that Dutch *huisartsen* have a unique relationship to their patients and a practice that is markedly different from their U.S. counterparts. In this chapter, we will talk about doctor-patient relationship, focusing on what *huisartsen* feel their role is at the end of life and in euthanasia discussions. *Huisartsen* participate in euthanasia because they feel their role at the end is beneficial to their patients and their patient's families. Chapter 4 looks at how *huisartsen* employ ideal concepts of death to shape the end-of-life experience. Finally, we will take a closer look at how *huisartsen* are contributing to the maintenance of Dutch life by talking euthanasia with their patients and their patients' families.

Chapter 5 is about the role and perspective of the dying individual. This chapter begins with the story of one man with HIV/AIDS, reflecting on what it means to die in the context of his life, his upbringing and his marriage to an American man. Death in many places is probably one of the single-most feared events of anyone's life. This chapter looks at how a few Dutch people experienced this time and what resources and ideals individuals employ to negotiate end of life. Chapter 5 looks at what form the Dutch penchant for control has taken in The Netherlands and how participation in euthanasia talk helps keep dying individuals connected to social life.

Chapter 6 focuses on the role and perspective of the family, a group largely overlooked in Dutch policy, but quite prevalent in the practice of euthanasia and end-of-life care in The Netherlands. The chapter begins with the story of a husband who reflects on the life he shared with his wife before her euthanasia death. Using this story and others as example, Chapter 6 explores the important role families assume in euthanasia talk and end-of-life care. Compared to the family experience in the U.S., the Dutch family-doctor relationship is much more cooperative. I will explore the nature of the family-doctor-state relationships in Chapter 6 and how these relationships are impacting the management of memories and relationships for families at the end of Dutch life.

This book is not, however, just a Dutch story. It is also a story about what the Dutch can teach other countries, particularly the U.S., about end-of-life care and policies. Part III opens up the analysis to look at Dutch and U.S. policies from a larger cross-cultural perspective. Chapter 7 examines what may be gained from insight into the Dutch experience. Here I look closely at how euthanasia and other end-of-life policies and practices are embedded in the Dutch and American health care systems. I also explore in greater detail the link that euthanasia and assisted dying have shared with concepts of suicide and I look at how ideals of death are employed in the face of bodily decline, social loss and as a mechanism for staving off social death. Headlines such as, "They Pretended They Were God" (Griffin and Johnston 2006) and "License to Kill" (Smith 2001) periodically fuel the fear that once the U.S. takes a step towards legalizing euthanasia, people will die not of their own free will. In Chapter 7 I will discuss the subtle, yet powerful cultural differences between these two societies to find out how differing relationships to family, nature, God and society are impacting end of life. Finally, I will conclude Chapter 7 with a discussion of lessons learned, possible policy implications for the U.S. based on empirical evidence of end-of-life policy and practice from The Netherlands.

PART I

Euthanasia in Perspective

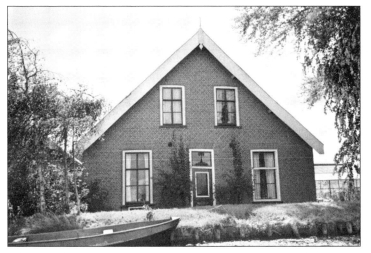

A home in the Dutch countryside. Photo credit: Frances Norwood

"*Slaap Lekker*" (Sleep Well)

I arrive at Dr. Maas' office a little after 2:00 in the afternoon.[1] *He is in with someone, so I sit in the waiting room until almost 3 o'clock. The Dutch are usually sticklers for time, so I am thinking maybe she did cancel. Dr. Maas finally waves me into his office and I sit there as he does some last minute preparations. On his desk is a box, which I*

---

1. All names and identifying information in this book have been changed to protect the confidentiality of participants. The events, however, are real and occurred in the city of Amsterdam or in a cluster of small towns outside of Amsterdam between the years 1999 and 2001.

assume carry the drugs that will end Marike van der Horst's life. Dr. Maas comes back in and asks me how my day was. "Het was anders *(It was different),*" *I said. For me too, he said. He sits down and opens the box to show me the drugs. He has more than he needs in case something goes wrong. In the box are two large bottles of Nesdonal (20 ml each) which will put her to sleep and six bottles of Pavulon (4 mg each) that, he says, are for "stopping her muscles." We head to the car and I ask why we are running late. He says that he spoke with Mr. van der Horst this morning and the family wanted to move it up to 3:30 p.m. Dr. Maas has already contacted the coroner, so they are all set for 3:30. Marike [pronounced MaREEkah] van der Horst was* "onrustig *(restless, agitated)*" *last night. Why, I ask, does she still want it? Yes, he says, she still wants to go through with it.*

We arrive and Maarten, her son, lets us in. The whole family is there: Marike and her husband, Joop [pronounced YOHP]; their grown children (Olv, Maarten and Frije [pronounced FRAYah]); their spouses; and another couple, family friends from down the street. Dr. Maas goes around the room, shaking hands and saying hello to everyone and I follow suit. Mr. van der Horst tells us they have decided to have only immediate family by her bedside when the time comes and the others will wait outside.

Dr. Maas goes to Mrs. van der Horst in the bed and asks if she knows why he is here. "No," *she says, confused then,* "yes." *(She's on large doses of morphine at this point).* "Are you sure?" *he asks.* "Ja, zeker *(Yes, certain),*" *she replies.* "She is certain," *her husband echoes. Dr. Maas, addressing everyone now, says all right, I will give you a needle and the first one will make you sleep and you won't wake up again. I'll prepare it in the kitchen, he says, and let you say goodbye while we do that.*

We go to the kitchen and I hear family members sniffling, crying and saying goodbye. Dr. Maas prepares the syringes, fumbling a bit as he goes, showing me for the first time that he too is nervous. I look out the kitchen window and see the extended family milling around in the back yard now, hugging each other and crying, and some looking into the window to see what we are doing.

We return to the living room, Dr. Maas with his black bag and syringes. Dr. Maas has Mr. van der Horst and the boys move the bed out from the wall so that everyone can have a place at her bedside. I feel nervous and numb, and very much like an intruder. Frije is really crying now, as she and her father take up positions at the head of her mother's bed. Olv and Maarten come to stand next to them, family on one side as Dr. Maas and I go to stand on the other side of the bed; Dr. Maas near her arm and I at her head. Family members are all holding each other and Joop is holding his wife's hand, everyone is sniffling or crying softly as Marike van der Horst says, "Het is best. Het is het beste zo. (It is best. It is for the best)." The family tells her to "slaap lekker, slaap lekker, mam (sleep well, sleep well, mom)." Dr. Maas tries for a vein on her arm and loses it then has me go get his second bag from the kitchen. My tears clear as Dr. Maas gives me something to focus on—getting his bag quickly. He finds a second vein and I see her blood flow into the tube he places there to hold the vein. Mrs. van der Horst is still saying that it is for the best as Dr. Maas inserts the first syringe. He fumbles a bit as he attempts to remove the needle, which is no longer necessary because of the tube holding her vein. "Slaap lekker, mam," I hear again as I watch Dr. Maas push the plunger on the syringe and look up in time to see Joop staring into his wife's eyes, gently rubbing her face. Within seconds she closes her eyes and her mouth falls slightly open. She doesn't move, blink, twitch or noticeably breathe again, and the cries get louder for a moment as she falls into asleep.

Seconds pass. Dr. Maas touches her eyelashes and she doesn't move. He empties the contents of the second syringe. I hear Joop say as he does it, "it's good" and "it is for the best." Dr. Maas pushes the plunger on the third syringe as I hear Joop van der Horst say, "It was enough;" and "It was too early, too early." "Ja (Yes)," Dr. Maas says, agreeing with him.

We wait, watching her for any sign. Dr. Maas breaks the moment, sending me for his stethoscope, which I get and pass to him. He checks with his fingers on the inside of her wrist for her pulse and uses the stethoscope to listen to her heart. She isn't breathing, he tells us, but her heart is still beating and I notice how the mood seems to lift when he explains things. We go back to watching and waiting, interrupted only by sniffling noses and family hugs. She doesn't move. It's a strange waiting that stretches the somber mood, until it feels no longer real. She's not breathing, her heart still beats and yet she looks the same— asleep. We wait, probably not more than 4 or 5 minutes, and then Dr. Maas checks her pupils by lifting her eyelids between forefinger and thumb. She is dilated, he tells us, and signals that it is over.

CHAPTER 2

MAKING A DISCOURSE[2]

Making the distinction between euthanasia (talk) and euthanasia (death) is critical to understanding just what the Dutch are doing at the end-of-life. In the preceding excerpt, we are introduced to Marike van der Horst in the final moments of what was a fairly brief illness episode compared to most patients with whom I worked. The above excerpt describes one euthanasia death that occurred in The Netherlands in 2001 and it is the "story" of euthanasia that tends to receive the most attention in the media (CNN 1998; Langley 2003; NYT 2001; NYT 2005; Okie 2002; SFC 2001) and by those from around the world who debate the Dutch experience with euthanasia (Foley and Hendin 2002; Have and Welie 2005; Klijn, et al. 2001; Ost 2003; Quill and Battin 2004; Thomasma and Graber 1990). It is not, however, the story of euthanasia most common in The Netherlands where euthanasia most often occurs as a dialogue between doctors, patients and families and not as a life-ending act. In 2001, for example, of those who initiated a request for euthanasia with their physician (which includes those who initiated requests in the event of a future serious illness), approximately 1 in 10 died a euthanasia death and two-fifths of those who made "concrete" requests (requests typically made after serious illness was diagnosed) died by euthanasia or assisted suicide (Wal, et al. 2003:46). By 2005, less than 1 in 10 who initiated requests and only one-third who made concrete requests died by euthanasia or assisted suicide. See Table 2.1.

---

2. Portions of this chapter were reprinted with permission by Taylor & Francis, Inc. (Norwood 2007).

Table 2.1 Percentage and Number of Euthanasia and
Physician-Assisted Suicide (PAS) Deaths in
The Netherlands, 1990–2005

	1990	1995	2001	2005
Termination of life on request	1.9%	2.6%	2.8%	1.8%
Euthanasia	1.7%	2.4%	2.6%	1.7%
PAS	0.2%	0.2%	0.2%	0.1%
Estimated euthanasia/PAS deaths*	2,448	3,528	3,931	2,455
Requests for euthanasia/PAS**				
Initiated requests	25,100	34,500	34,700	28,600
Concrete requests	8,900	9,700	9,700	8,400
Ratio of euthanasia/PAS deaths to***				
Initiated requests	9.8%	10.2%	11.3%	8.6%
Concrete requests	27.5%	36.4%	40.5%	29.2%
Total deaths	128,824	135,675	140,377	136,402

* Estimated by multiplying percent of euthanasia/PAS deaths by total deaths.

** Requests are distinguished by "initiated requests" include requests made in the final days, weeks and months before death as well as requests made in the event of future illness and "concrete requests" for those requests that typically occur once an irreversible illness has been diagnosed and death in the coming days, weeks or months is imminent.

*** Estimated by dividing total number of euthanasia and PAS requests by number of initiated and concrete requests.

Source: (Onwuteaka-Philipsen, et al. 2007:100, 108; Wal, et al. 2003:46). These estimates use the death certificate portion of the van der Wal and van der Maas studies because of evidence that suggests these are the most reliable estimates (Griffiths, et al. 2008:149). For more on the results of the longitudinal study by Van der Wal and Van der Maas available in the English language, see (Heide, et al. 2003; Heide, et al. 2007; Maas, et al. 1996).

What is 'euthanasia talk'? On one level, it is what it suggests, a discussion for the purpose of planning a person's euthanasia death. It is also, however, a product of a *discourse*, a cultural form that shapes the production, practice and interpretation of life and end-of-life. Discourse is a concept that has gained increasing attention in anthropology following the work of Foucault (1972; 1991), Laclau and Mouffe (1985), Habermas (1992; 1996) and Bourdieu (1992). In a sense, much of what is produced today in anthropology is loosely inclusive of a concept of 'discourse' as a medium link-ing knowledge, power, and practice (Behar and Gordon 1995; Clifford and Marcus 1986; Faubion 1993; Franklin and Lock 2003; Haraway 2004; Harding 2000).

Probably one of the most influential theorists currently on the topic of discourse is Michel Foucault (Foucault 1972; Foucault 1978; Foucault 1991). Foucault's concept of discourse changes somewhat throughout his writings (Paras 2006), thus to be specific I will focus on the way he talks about discourse in relation to the production of knowledge and power in *The Archaeology of Knowledge* (1972) and how he delineates the structure of discourse in "Politics and the Study of Discourse" (1991). Foucault defines discourse as a "an individualized group of statements" and as a "regulated practice that accounts for a certain number of statements" (Foucault 1972:79–80). Thus, discourse can initially be understood as both a grouping of statements and the rules by which those statements are formed. Foucault's concept of discourse is not just about language or the structure of language; however, it is about a discursive practice based on rules of exclusion that allow or disallow participation by individual subjects. Individuals may assume existing subject positions (sometimes successfully, sometimes unsuccessfully), using the language of various discourses in dominant circulation. Discourses in turn limit what can be spoken, what is constituted as taboo, what is held in collective conscience, what is reconstituted from the past, and who in society has access.

In sum, discourse exists in language and in practice (1) as collections of statements, (2) as rules for the formation of those statements, and (3) as practices of circulation and exclusion. The consequences of discourse are enormous. Foucault writes, "in every society the production of discourse is at once controlled, selected, organised and redistributed according to a certain number of procedures, whose role is to avert its power and its dangers, to cope with chance events, [and] to evade its ponderous, awesome materiality" (Foucault 1972:216). Discourse produces knowledge in forms that we come to think of as normative (as understood) and, in doing so, discourse obscures its very nature—that it is a cultural form that shapes the way we think, feel and act (Foucault 1972:115; Foucault 1991:58–60).

I am suggesting that in The Netherlands a discourse has emerged that dominates end of life discussions and practices; this discourse takes the form of euthanasia talk. Thomas Scheff (1990) suggests that end-of-life around the world is marked by an inherent drive people have to maintain sociality, to maintain a social identity and social relationships. We know that the experience of death and dying has changed over time and that what was formerly a typically short-term event has through the many advances in medical knowledge and treatments been extended, marked more often by long periods of decline and social losses (Lynn 2004:4–31).[3] Seale (1998) suggests that in modern times there are at least two ways that sociality is maintained in modern-day death and dying. First, dying persons may participate in a kind of "revivalist discourse,"[4] a socio-therapeutic narrative whereby their social losses are transformed into something meaningful and affirming. Second, dying persons may seek euthanasia or assisted suicide, to have the time of bio-

---

3. This new dying trajectory only applies in countries where health care and public health measures have advanced and are readily available to a majority of the population. The U.S. is a strange anomaly compared to most "Western" countries where health care tends to be made available on a universal access basis. The current U.S. health care system does have aspects of universal access for limited segments of the population, including Medicare which partially covers approximately four-fifths of those who are sick and dying and Medicaid which covers those who live in poverty or who have been made impoverished as a result of their illness (Lynn 2004:28–31). Health care reform towards a system of universal access in the U.S. is long overdue.

4. Foucault and Seale use the term "discourse" in very different ways. For Foucault it is a theoretical construct that he uses to understand what we see, hear, and experience. For Seale, it is a term that is used to delineate a more limited practice, a kind of shared collection of statements. In order to avoid confusion, in this book I will be using Foucault's concept of discourse and only the content of ideas expressed by Seale's use of the term.

logical death (death of the body) adjusted to coincide more closely with social death (death of the social being) (Seale 1998:7–8).

Both Foucault and Seale provide valuable clues to understanding the Dutch experience at the end of life. Foucault offers the framework for how to see past the obvious to the more subtle underpinnings of Dutch end of life and Seale offers clues to understanding the content of euthanasia talk, suggesting that end-of-life practices may be a way the Dutch have developed to stave off social death. In this chapter, we will explore the structural and cultural underpinnings of euthanasia talk, which will allow us to better understand just what Dutch people are doing when they invoke euthanasia at the end of life. Our story begins with an ethnographic excerpt of one woman and a description of the discussions and practices that are more typically experienced by those who initiate a request for euthanasia in The Netherlands.

"*Niks Meer Aan te Doen*" (Nothing More to Do)

Ms. Els Bosma was first diagnosed with rectal cancer in 1994. She was treated with radiation in 1994 then again in 1998 when a second mass was found in her lower intestine. By September 2000, at age 59, Ms. Bosma was told there was "niks meer aan te doen" *(nothing more to do). Her treatment phase was over. In September, Ms. Bosma came home from the hospital with the intent to die there.*

Els Bosma was an independent woman, never married, but with a large circle of friends who visited often, a sister who came by daily and an elderly father who was fairly religious, sometimes confused and very distraught about losing his daughter. Ms. Bosma was a schoolteacher most of her life and told me she liked her life. I found her to be a matter-of-fact type person, direct and to the point when she was not talking about really difficult issues. Her huisarts *saw her as a private person and, while he had a personable relationship with her, she tended to hold him at arm's length, maintaining a social distance that he found difficult at times. She was the first person that I interviewed in this study and I was nervous with her, scared to overstay my welcome or to ask questions that might upset her. At the end of our first interview she told me I needed to ask my questions, otherwise, she said, how would I ever get the answers? I liked her style.*

I first met Ms. Bosma in September, during a planning meeting at her home scheduled by her huisarts, *Dr. Muller. She was there, thin and tall with short brown hair and casual clothes, half sitting on the couch where she had been resting earlier as evidenced by a pillow and blanket. She sat with one hip raised and leaning on the armrest so that she could sit sideways. Clearly sitting was uncomfortable for her. The room was typical of Dutch homes, a small living room with a large picture window overlooking the back garden. With her in the living room was her sister (Janneke [pronounced YAHNahkah]), their elderly father, her sister's female partner, the nurse (Marjan [pronounced MARyahn]) from* Thuiszorg,[5] *the national homecare service, Dr. Muller and myself. We shuffled chairs and people in this small space and negotiated the pouring of tea before Dr. Muller began the meeting. He asks if everyone knows what we are here for and reminds us that there is "*niks meer aan te doen.*" Ms. Bosma says yes and then someone asks her father if he understands. He says yes, she has cancer and she's home now. Ms. Bosma says she's here because she doesn't want to be in the hospital anymore, the hospital tires her out. Dr. Muller says he understands and he and Marjan begin to lay out what types of services are now available to Ms. Bosma. The meeting continues, meandering back and forth between issues of sleeping, eating and service options.*

---

5. *Thuiszorg* is literally translated to mean "Homecare." It is the national organization which provides home care services free of charge or on a sliding scale fee to all Dutch citizens. Services include nursing and personal care assistance up to four times a day in the home, including an all-night overnight service. *Thuiszorg* employees set out meals, provide all manner of hygiene and nursing care, and even provide a weekly cleaning service for the home. While in The Netherlands, I also conducted participant observation with personal care assistants with *Amsterdam Thuiszorg.*

I didn't see Ms. Bosma again until a house call with her huisarts *the following week. By then her living room had been transformed into the sick room that I got very used to seeing in the homes I visited. The couch had been replaced with an adjustable hospital bed overlooking the back garden and her side table was cluttered with tissues, untouched sandwich halves, medicine bottles and drinking cups with straws. During this visit, Ms. Bosma was having a lot of trouble with nausea — gagging intermittingly while we talked to her — and I could smell a sickly sweet smell from the tube that drained the abscess in her lower intestines. Dr. Muller asks if she might want to go to the hospital and she says she doesn't want to go, but she's not sure. She is worried that her specialists are not treating her. She also says her friends don't seem to know how to deal with her changes. They bring things she used to like and she knows they are just trying to be helpful, so she pretends she still likes it. She smiles a sweet shrugging smile and we smile back.*

Three days later we have our first interview alone together and I find out that Ms. Bosma did decide to go the hospital, but there was nothing they could do for her. I asked if she would go to the hospital again in the future and she says "definitely no more." Knowing my research topic, she offers that she has read information on euthanasia but knows it's not for her. Like many others, however, Ms. Bosma has misconceptions about how euthanasia actually works. She thinks, for example, that there is a mandatory 5-day waiting period between deciding for euthanasia and receiving it.[6] How could you schedule something like that, she asks. Also she has already experienced how bad it can get and she has morphine for the pain so she doesn't need euthana-

---

6. Ms. Bosma, like many Dutch people I met, seemed to be slightly confused about the specifics of the regulations for euthanasia. There is no mandatory five day waiting period, but doctor's do attempt to stretch out the time between a request for euthanasia and a euthanasia death. I found the most common misunderstanding about euthanasia to be that once you decided you were ready for euthanasia, it was your decision alone to make and it could occur when you wanted it (e.g., that day). This is not the case.

sia. She tells me she isn't scared about the future, because she's had a good life.

At the end of October, Ms. Bosma again went to the hospital to have the drain to her intestines checked. At that time, and unbeknownst to us, her specialist raised euthanasia as a "treatment" option. This I came to find out was not done frequently in The Netherlands, but was also not unusual. The next day Dr. Muller and I pay a house call and find Ms. Bosma in a somber mood, propped up in bed smoking a cigarette and staring into the back garden. Janneke, her sister, is there. Dr. Muller asks if she's going to put the cigarette out and she does without turning to face us. Dr. Muller gets up to stand at the foot of her bed to better see her face which is still turned toward the garden. She tells Dr. Muller she was in the hospital because the last five days or so she's been having bad pain and can feel another tumor growing. She reaches down to her abdominal area to show us, coughs, and immediately cries out in pain. "Ow, ow, ow," she says wincing and we all pause. She is quiet for a while then apologizes, "sorry." "No, don't be sorry," Dr. Muller says looking concerned. She's scheduled to go back to the hospital on Monday, she says, but she thinks it is inoperable. Dr. Muller asks if they are going to change her drain. She doesn't know but she's had a fever.

"You have three options," Dr. Muller tells her, "one, they can change your drain; two …"

"Euthanasia," she interrupts. She's talked to the specialist about it and doesn't know if she can decide five days in advance but she has a lot of pain and good days and bad days, and.…

Dr. Muller sits down in a chair at the foot of her bed and I look around to see her sister silent, sitting in the chair in the corner. Dr. Muller listens, pauses, then says yes, euthanasia is a possibility and she can have the specialist do it in the hospital or he can do it for her here at home. She should think about who she is most comfortable with and it won't make a difference with him. Ms. Bosma's sister says, no, they don't know the hospital doctor so well and Ms. Bosma adds that she doesn't want to go to the hospital. First, he says, she must have several discussions about it with him and also with her family. That is really important, he emphasizes, that you talk to your family.

Does your father know you're thinking about this? No, she hasn't told him. He can help with that if she wants. He can, for example, schedule a family meeting to talk about it with him. Next, she must make her written euthanasia declaration, and make plans for it but that doesn't mean she has to go through with it. Some patients just make the plan, then things progress and they don't choose euthanasia, he says. Her sister asks if they have to wait another five days if they cancel the euthanasia. No, that's not necessary. There is no five-day waiting period, it's just that you have to plan it. Finally, a second doctor must come see her to talk to her about it. Dr. Muller asks if her sister has any questions. No. Ms. Bosma? Questions? No. He goes on to talk about medications, then asks Ms. Bosma if he should make a note that this is her official request for going forward with euthanasia planning? Yes, she says adamantly. We leave and before biking in different directions—he to his next appointment and me to mine, we share our surprise at the sudden request for euthanasia and Dr. Muller tells me that her father is really religious and she doesn't want to be a disappointment to him.

Two days later, I meet with Ms. Bosma again for an interview and we begin by talking about how she's feeling. We talk about pain and she says she hasn't had much pain in her life, and now she has some but she takes the painkillers and she doesn't mind them but it does make her fuzzy. We're talked about feeling good and the false optimism she gets, like when she felt good last week. She says she feels "akelig," it's a "yucky sick" feeling, she explains, not really pain, but yucky sick. She sleeps a lot and likes that because it makes her feel better when she wakes up. Things have been up and down, she says, fever at night and problems with the drain burning and feeling hot. The fever, she says, makes her feel sicker. I ask if she thinks that between Dr. Muller and the hospital they can fix that.

Ms. Bosma: I think so, yes. Tomorrow I have an appointment because I want to set in motion plans for euthanasia. The doctor from the hospital said that too, that otherwise I'm pretty healthy and this could last a long time. So he said, we've done all we can do and I find this a good reason to say, now we can't cure you and you won't remain healthy, it can only get worse and worse.

Frances: So you choose for euthanasia on account of your talk with the hospital doctor and because it might last a long time?

Ms. Bosma: Yes, exactly. No, but I don't know when it will happen. That could be well down the road. It's dependent on the situation and how sick I feel or not. But if I really feel ill, then I can't keep going. Then it may be too late to bring it [euthanasia] up.

A month after our first interview together, Ms. Bosma explains to me that she is clear now on how euthanasia works. Before she thought that once you set a date, you had to go through with it. "But now I understand that you don't have to. It works another way. If you change your mind and say no, then you don't have to go through everything all over again to set a new date." She is still unsure, though, about being able to say okay, I'm going to die on this day. The fact that she can do it at home with her huisarts is also important. She doesn't want to go back to the hospital anymore.

The following day, I am back at Ms. Bosma's for the family meeting that Dr. Muller has scheduled to discuss her euthanasia request. It is a typically wet Dutch day and I arrive soaked to the skin on my bicycle in spite of all the gear I regularly wear to hold the water at bay. I wait for Dr. Muller under an overhang outside Ms. Bosma's door and watch through blurry, wet glasses as he pulls up nonchalantly on his bicycle. He's wearing his leather today and somehow arrives Dutch rumpled but relatively unscathed by the rain. Janneke lets us in and I must peel wet layers off in the foyer. How do you do it, I ask him, how do you stay dry? Dr. Muller smiles at me that amused and sympathetic smile reserved for us foreigners.

Everyone is here: Ms. Bosma, her father, Janneke and her partner. The room feels a little tense this time, with Ms. Bosma smoking, propped up in her bed and us trying to arrange ourselves once again in chairs around the small, crowded room. Tea is poured and Dr. Muller begins the meeting by asking what the main complaint today is. Ms. Bosma starts to answer and then stops, staring out into the back garden. Dr. Muller prompts her by summarizing some things (not mentioning euthanasia yet) and she again just sits there, not responding. He asks if she has something she wants to say to everyone and she starts to speak, but it's broken speech, nothing

*about euthanasia, and again she falls quiet. I watch her and no-
tice the glazed morphine stare of someone on high doses of painkiller
and assume that her drugs are affecting things today. We wait. Dr.
Muller starts again, explaining that he was here earlier this week
and talked about the possibility of euthanasia, which is why everyone is assembled today. Mr. Bosma, tall and thin like his daughter, speaks up, volunteering that they have talked about it. And
how do you feel about it, Dr. Muller asks. Mr. Bosma starts to answer then begins to cry. He says he understands but would be more
comfortable with it if he knew she only had a short time to live.
Dr. Muller says it is important that he respect her decision — that
is important. Mr. Bosma nods yes through his tears. The doctor
says it is her decision but it is also important to talk about it with
family and friends. Janneke says she understands. Dr. Muller turns
again to Ms. Bosma and asks her why does she want euthanasia?
She stares. What is so terrible, he asks? No answer. Her sister offers that maybe it's because she is sick all day long. Ms. Bosma says
no, that's not it. "Oh, I'm not right," she replies. Silence. Dr. Muller
presses, asking her what makes it so difficult to talk about. No answer. Is it because we're all here, her sister's partner asks. No, she
answers. Well, says Dr. Muller, you'll have to think about that because when the SCEA[7] doctor comes, that's what he'll need to know.
Janneke agrees, yes, you'll have to think about that, and suggests
that maybe the painkillers are a problem today. Dr. Muller — addressing everyone now — explains that the first step is to make a eu-*

---

7. *Steun en Consultatie bij Euthanasie in Amsterdam* [Support and Consultation for Euthanasia in Amsterdam] (SCEA) is an organization of and
for doctors in the greater Amsterdam area who have questions about euthanasia or need to schedule an independent, second opinion for a euthanasia or assisted suicide case. It was created in 1997 in collaboration with
the *Koninklijke Nederlandsche Maatschappij tot bevordering der Geneeskunst*
[Royal Dutch Society for the Promotion of Health] (KNMG) and the *Amsterdamse Huisartsenvereniging* [Amsterdam General Practice Association]
(AHV) (Onwuteaka-Philipsen and Wal 1998).

8. The *Nederlandse Vereniging voor een Vrijwillig Levenseinde* [Dutch Association for Voluntary End-of-life] (NVVE) was formed in 1973 by a

thanasia declaration, which is from Ms. Bosma and states in writing that her decision is voluntary. The Dutch Association for Voluntary End-of-Life (NVVE)[8] can help them with that. Then a second doctor will come to talk to her. On the technical side, they must decide whether to have a drink or a needle but that is the technical side. Half of the people who talk about it don't do it because they choose not to or because sickness overtakes them. What we are talking about, he says, is just preparing for it. Outside, Dr. Muller tells me, "It is doubtful now."

On a house call the next day, Dr. Muller receives a copy of the signed euthanasia declaration from Janneke with signatures from Ms. Bosma and the whole family.[9] The next day, Ms. Bosma checks to see that her declaration is sufficient. It is and now, Dr. Muller states, the preparation has been done. Now you must tell me when you want to have it, when for you the time is near. Not until then, will the second doctor come. Well, she says, it will depend on what happens with the drain and that it is difficult to know. What about the pain, Dr. Muller asks as they move on to other topics.

Two months after her terminal diagnosis and two weeks after her initial request for euthanasia, Els Bosma died of her disease. She didn't ask for euthanasia again, and in the last days before her death, Dr. Muller said he pretty much knew the euthanasia was not going to go through. She declined quickly at the end. She complained of pain, high fever, benauwdheid *(tightness in the chest or anxiety),*[10] *and*

---

group of doctors following the *Postma* case. Today, the NVVE has a membership of over 100,000. The goals of the NVVE are to advance "social acceptance of the existing legal possibilities towards a free choice on the end of life;" "social acceptance of legal possibilities that are not currently within the scope of existing regulations;" and the "recognition of free choice [at] the end of life" as a human right (NVVE 2004).

   9. All of the euthanasia declarations that I read were signed by family members in addition to the individual requesting the euthanasia.

   10. *Benauwdheid* is a term used by patients and physicians to describe a symptom that has both physical and mental attributes. It is translated to mean "tightness of the chest," "closeness, stuffiness," "fear, anxiety," and "distress" (Hannay and Schrama 1996:81).

was in and out of consciousness. I asked Dr. Muller afterward what he felt was her main reason for requesting euthanasia. He said, to prepare for a future that might be worse. He was disturbed that she couldn't talk much about her request and thought that it was because she wasn't ready to leave her family. If her request had gone further, he said, he would have needed her to talk more openly about why she wanted it. According to Marjan, it was a good experience for Thuiszorg employees. Ms. Bosma wanted to stay at home and with only her sister to help, Thuiszorg *was able to grant her wish. Like Dr. Muller, Marjan was skeptical about her euthanasia request, saying that it seemed to come more from the hospital doctor than from Ms. Bosma. Ms. Bosma, she said, was happy with life and wanted to live it.*

An End-of-Life Discourse

I highlight Ms. Bosma's experience because compared to Ms. Van der Horst's euthanasia death that opens this section, it is the experience that is most common to the people I met and the stories they told. *Euthanasia talk* is the term I am using to describe the dialogue that typically occurs among dying persons, family members and their physician (in this study, the *huisarts*) following a request for euthanasia. Euthanasia talk, itself, is not a discourse, but it is a product of an end-of-life discourse in the Foucauldian sense of the term. Euthanasia talk, I found, consisted of a number of regularities, which I saw repeated in 25 intensive case studies and in observations and testimonials from countless other patients, family members, and physicians included in this study. Foucault suggests that discourse is a discursive formation that exists (1) as collections of statements, (2) as rules for the formulation of those statements and (3) as practices of circulation and exclusion. In the following section, we will explore just what Foucault means by that and how euthanasia talk may be evidence for an end-of-life discourse that occurs in The Netherlands. First, however, I want to set a little of the cultural context for euthanasia talk.

A Practice Based in *Overleg* (Consultation)

In the next chapter, I will explore in great detail the cultural and historical context that makes up end-of-life discourses around the world, and in particular in The Netherlands. Here, however, it is appropriate to introduce the reader to the Dutch practice of *overleg*, which defines much of Dutch interaction, including Dutch medical practice and euthanasia talk. *Overleggen* is translated to mean "to consider, consult, or confer" (Hannay and Schrama 1996:609). The literal translation of the word, however, is not adequate to describe the nuance and the prevalence of this practice in Dutch life. It is a commonly used process in The Netherlands with a number of unspoken rules whereby consensus building occurs and decisions get made. It is used in politics, in business and in many other realms of social life. Dutch cultural historian Han van der Horst describes the practice of *overleg* (consultation):

> The literal translation 'consultation' does not embrace the full meaning of the term in Dutch. [*Overleg*] is a form of group communication which aims not so much at reaching a decision as giving the parties involved the opportunity to exchange information. The Dutch spend many of their working hours in *overleg*. This means that they are discussing the state of affairs with their colleagues. They describe in detail the activities they are engaged in and the rest of the group are, in principle, entitled to make comments or ask questions (Horst 2001:170).

In Dutch medical practice, *overleg* requires a more equalized power differential between patients and *huisartsen*, encouraging *huisartsen* to facilitate health (not proscribe it) and focusing medical practice on discussion over action. A typical office visit, for example, begins in the *spreekkamer* (or consultation room) seated across from or cattycorner to the *huisarts* who is always dressed in regular street clothes, not the white coat and stethoscope necklace attire of their U.S. counterparts. Most of the visit is spent discussing the problem, including any 'psychosocial issues' that the *huisarts* deems relevant, such as stress on the job or problems in the marriage. Examination of the body always occurs second and sometimes not at all in a separate room called the *onderzoekskamer* (or examination room). In a typical morning of office visits, the *huisarts* may use the examination room in less than half of all visits (Norwood 2005:100). Euthanasia practice also follows this model. While the *huisarts* always takes charge of the discussion and ultimately the decision to perform euthanasia or not, euthanasia talk is based on a relatively flat power differential where all participants are encouraged to participate in the dialogue, reflecting on how they feel about the request for euthanasia.

A Collection of Statements

The practice of *overleg* provides the context for taking a closer look at the structure of euthanasia talk. My research revealed uniformity to euthanasia talk that conforms to at least five measurable stages.[11] These stages can be identified by distinct sections within euthanasia discussions that are typically bound at the front end by the patient initiating a move forward in the planning process and at the back end by the *huisarts* pausing the discussion, leaving the onus on the patient to re-initiate euthanasia discussions. These uniform stages plot the course of euthanasia talk as they form a collection of statements intended for the general purpose of planning someone's euthanasia death. The stages include: (1) initial euthanasia requests, (2) written declarations, (3) second opinion appointment, (4) scheduling euthanasia, and (5)

---

11. If I could have found a way to track repeated requests, that would have been another "stage" in the euthanasia discussion. Because they occur often during the course of discussions, these were too difficult to track as their own separate stage.

euthanasia death. Figure 2.1 demonstrates the movement of 14 persons as they initiated and progressed through these five stages of euthanasia talk.

The five stages are as follows. First, there are initial verbal requests and written declarations that occur anywhere from years before death to weeks and days before death. These tend to be initiated at the first sign of serious illness, but can occur before that and well after that for a number of different reasons. Initial requests establish the first official evidence necessary for a "long standing" desire for euthanasia (as per Dutch regulations); they serve as insurance for an unknowable future; they establish a *huisarts'* willingness to perform euthanasia; they allow the *huisarts* an opportunity to communicate the formal and informal rules for euthanasia negotiations; and they allow the *huisarts* to clear up any misunderstandings about how euthanasia gets done. In Ms. Bosma's case, her initial request came relatively late in relation to her illness. Prior to her request she made it clear that euthanasia was not something she was interested in and this was her stance after many years living with cancer. Her request for euthanasia came well into her terminal phase

Figure 2.1 Five Stages of Euthanasia Talk (n=14)

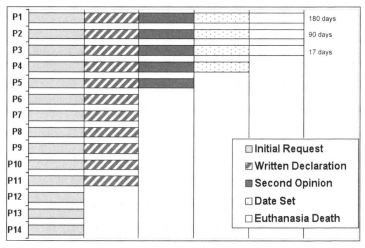

(which is not typical), raising some questions about the authenticity of her request with her *huisarts*. Turns out the suggestion for euthanasia did not come from Ms. Bosma herself, it came from her hospital specialist who suggested euthanasia as an end-of-life option. This is something that does occur, though somewhat infrequently in The Netherlands. Ms. Bosma knew that no discussion of euthanasia would proceed without an established official record of her request, so within days of her initial request, Ms. Bosma submitted her written declaration, confirming with her *huisarts* that it would be sufficient to proceed.

Initial requests for euthanasia open the dialogue and serve as a means for the *huisarts* to communicate his or her role, to clarify procedures, and to clear up any misunderstandings about how euthanasia works. Dr. Muller, like every other *huisartsen* with whom I worked, stressed the importance of discussing the request with him and with family members and explained that this was about planning for a euthanasia death, but not necessarily going through with it. This is what I heard every *huisarts* say. Dr. Muller also cleared up misunderstandings because although euthanasia is a common topic in public discourses, the details of the practice are not universally understood. No, it is not only the patient's choice, physicians must agree to perform euthanasia; no, you don't have to schedule your death five days in advance and; no, once you schedule euthanasia you do not have to go through with it. Finally, Dr. Muller communicated his role in the process. Euthanasia discussions are managed by *huisartsen*. Dr. Muller took it on himself to facilitate communication between Ms. Bosma and her father. It was he who called the family meeting and it was he who took charge of the content, speed, and trajectory of the discussions.

Requests (verbal and written) must be repeated and patients who do repeat their request are asked to explain why they want euthanasia over and over again. In Ms. Bosma's case, she was not able to articulate why she wanted it, causing her *huisarts* to pause the discussion after the written declaration and before the scheduling of a second opinion. The pause is critical. Like all other *huisartsen* with whom I worked, not one doctor said to a patient outright that they could not have euthanasia. Outright confrontation in the process of *overleg* is not part of the practice that is based in compromise (Horst 2001:167–181). Instead, *huisartsen* pause the process; they slow it down and wait it out. In Ms. Bosma's case, these pauses (without outright rejection of her request) allowed her to relax, knowing that *if* she wanted to proceed the door was still open. From the perspective of her *huisarts,* however, it was clear that there would need to be firmer evidence that the request was genuine and met both the proper legal requirements and his personal requirements to proceed.

Initial requests, written declarations and subsequent repeated requests are typically as far as most patients go in the stages of a euthanasia discussion. In my case study sample, only 5 of 14 initiated setting an appointment with a second physician to confirm that the request for euthanasia met legal regulations. The likelihood of a euthanasia death occurring goes up considerably once someone gets a second opinion. Of 5 who received a second opinion, 4 scheduled a date for euthanasia and 3 died euthanasia deaths. Most second opinion appointments occur within 24 to 48 hours of the euthanasia death and all must be appointments with a physician who is deemed "independent" of the first. For the *huisarts* to agree to schedule a second doctor, he or she must be sufficiently convinced that the request meets the policy regulations and his or her personal and professional limits of what constitutes a proper request. Once a second opinion is scheduled, however, there are still several events that can stop a euthanasia death from occurring. The patient must repeat their request to schedule a date for euthanasia (stage 4) and must typically repeat their reason for their request the day the date is scheduled (stage 5). If the individual changes their mind, they must be able to tell the *huisarts* or a family member (or at least hesitate like Ms. Bosma did when asked why they want the process to proceed causing the *huisarts* to once again halt the proceedings). Family holds the power to stop a euthanasia death by opposing it so strongly that the patient relents. Just as likely, however, the illness itself may stop a euthanasia death in these final stages by either proceeding so quickly that the patient dies or by going into some form of remission. Of five who reached the second opinion stage, three died euthanasia deaths, one woman died in her sleep the day of her second opinion appointment, and one woman cancelled her date with euthanasia due to pressure from her daughter.

The Rules: Inclusions to Euthanasia Talk

According to Foucault, discourse is both a collection of statements and the rules by which those statements are formed. In the case of euthanasia talk, there are formal, written rules that have developed over the course of more than 30 years of public dialogue and 20 years of legal practice. These rules currently exist in The Netherlands as the *Termination of Life on Request and Assisted Suicide (Review Procedures) Act* (The Act 2002). According to the Act, euthanasia and assisted suicide must always be performed by a physician who:

a. holds the conviction that the request by the patient was voluntary and well-considered,

b. holds the conviction that the patient's suffering was lasting and unbearable,

c. has informed the patient about the situation he was in and about his prospects,

d. and the patient holds the conviction that there was no other reasonable solution for the situation he was in,

e. has consulted at least one other, independent physician who has seen the patient and has given his written opinion on the requirements of due care, referred to in parts a–d, and

f. has terminated a life or assisted in a suicide with due care (Requirements for Due Care, Article 2, The Act 2002).

Beyond these formal rules, however, there exist a whole range of informal, mostly unspoken rules that shape the practice of euthanasia talk and euthanasia death. Looking closely at these formal and informal rules, we begin to see a practice that goes deeper than the obvious planning for euthanasia death.

The law requires physicians to take charge of euthanasia discussions. Under the law, only Dutch physicians may perform euthanasia or assisted suicide and the law is written with the focus on the role and responsibilities of the doctor. At the first mention of euthanasia, Dr. Muller firmly established himself as the person in charge of the discussion and no *huisarts* with whom I worked (regardless of personality) failed to take a leadership role in the progression of this discussion. While Ms. Bosma could always restart the dialogue, Dr. Muller took control of what topics were relevant to the discussion, how quickly the discussion progressed, and who was to be included. In spite of popular rhetoric which circulates to some degree in The Netherlands around an individual's right to choose (Chabot 2001:70), it is (in practice) the *physician's* right to manage euthanasia talk and (where needed) stall euthanasia death. *Huisartsen* are clearly in control of euthanasia talk and they see their role in these discussions as facilitators of the dying process.

Because euthanasia talk has come to be based in the cultural practice of *overleg* (consultation), it is critical for all involved that patients, families and *huisartsen* participate, which means that the person with the request must talk to family and their *huisarts* and discuss why they are considering euthanasia, what they fear, and what preferences they have for their end of life care. A byproduct of this communication, which occurs mostly according to informal rules for how a request gets considered, is that participants of the dialogue through the active roles they assume draw closer. Six of 10 *huisartsen* in my study described their most satisfying cases of euthanasia as ones in which the relationship with patients and/or families grew as a result of euthanasia discussions and/or euthanasia deaths. Patients and families, too, described a special bond that occurs with their *huisarts* when euthanasia is seriously considered.

One of the most prominent and prevalent activities that occurred in the course of euthanasia talk was the push by *huisartsen* for patients to discuss the reason and the meaning of their request with family and with their *huisarts*. While the law dictates that the request must be "well considered," it does not mention with whom or how. Nowhere in the law is there mention of family. Yet, informally, families assume an integral role in euthanasia discussions. Part of that may be because the unique style and structure of general practice in The Netherlands. Many *huisartsen* have known their patients for many years, often treating them, their children, and their children's children. But it is not just about the length of the relationship; it is about the quality and the nature of it. Compared to other physicians, *huisartsen* generally consider themselves a different breed of doctor. They pride themselves on being the doctor that treats the "whole" patient in the context of their illness, their daily stresses and their relationships (Groenewegen and Delnoij 1997; Muijsenbergh 2001). Changes have been occurring, however, that are impacting the nature of the *huisarts*-patient-family relationship and city *huisartsen*, especially, are feeling the impact as their patient populations grow to include more non-Dutch immigrants and more transitory patient populations.

Dr. Muller (like a growing number of his city counterparts) had not known Ms. Bosma that long and, in fact, expressed regret that he and Ms. Bosma did not draw into a closer relationship as a result of their euthanasia talks. While Ms. Bosma may have remained a little distant from her *huisarts*, Dr. Muller continued to follow informal patterns of euthanasia practice, orchestrating family and patient dialogues regarding Ms. Bosma's request. Dr. Muller's role as facilitator of family discussions (e.g., making sure that the father understood what his daughter was requesting and accepted, or at least respected, her decision) was typical for nearly every *huisarts* with whom I worked. It was not unusual, for example, for *huisartsen* to initiate contact (not at the patient's request) with estranged family members in the hopes of facilitating a reunion before death.

Consider Ms. Bosma's euthanasia request. For her, the tension was situated somewhere between her right to decide for herself what she wanted at the end of her life and the practical reality of anyone considering euthanasia. The reality is that most people do not make important (life and death) decisions without consideration of and in consultation with the people they care about. Ms. Bosma, like the large majority in my study, made her request in the context of familial and societal relationships.

The Rules: Exclusions to Euthanasia Talk

Foucault suggests that discourse functions on the basis of circulation and exclusion, limiting what can be said, what is constituted as taboo, and who within any given society has access (Foucault 1991:59–60). The focus on exclusions is important because it would not be accurate to suggest that what Dutch people do when they engage in euthanasia talk is seamless or always works toward cohesive social bonding (Durkheim 1912; Durkheim 1951). On the contrary, euthanasia talk (in practice) is complex and there are participants who function on the borders of this discourse and others that tend to get excluded from it based on (1) their unwillingness to participate, (2) their inability to function according to the formal and informal rules for engagement, or (3) characteristics of their case that are used by others to exclude them.

First, there are those who for religious or other reasons do not consider euthanasia an option. In the 1970s, Europe experienced sharp rates of decline in church attendance and affiliation, and The Netherlands, in particular, experienced some of the highest rates of secularization (Becker and Vink 1994; Shetter 1987:174). Even so, there are still sections of the country where religion has maintained a presence and there are those throughout the country who continue to oppose euthanasia based on their religious beliefs. Ms. Bosma's father was considered quite "religious" and was probably the biggest roadblock to her request for euthanasia, next to her own ambivalence.

Of those who do wish to participate in euthanasia talk, there are informal rules that must be addressed in order for someone to properly engage in this discourse. If someone fails to conform to these unwritten rules, it tends to raise what I call "red flags" (concerns) for *huisartsen. Huisartsen* react by slowing down the process or encouraging further dialogue around the topic of concern. Characteristics that most often get potential participants excluded from euthanasia talk are absence of participating family members or conflict that has not been addressed within the family, being too pushy or asking for euthanasia the wrong way, having an illness or disease that is non-specific or non-somatic (such as old age or psychological in origin), or exhibiting signs of untreatable depression.

In Ms. Bosma's case, she was not going to receive euthanasia unless she changed how she answered the question, "why?" Her hesitation to answer the question on multiple occasions and the fact that the request did not come from her initially all raised enough concern for Dr. Muller to stall movement toward euthanasia death. All patients are required in the course of a euthanasia discussion to communicate their wishes. In order to move their request forward, patients must repeatedly initiate requests for euthanasia and they must be able to respond when they are asked to explain why they want it. That explanation needs to meet not only formal rules, but informal rules for how to ask for euthanasia, which Ms. Bosma's request did not. Through her request for euthanasia, Ms. Bosma communicated to her family and Dr. Muller her fear of dying in too much pain and suffering, perhaps some fear of an unknowable future, and her need for some assurance that if it got worse she would have an option. At the same time, however, her inability to discuss the reason for her request communicated her reluctance to go through with it. Euthanasia was not really something she had considered for herself previously (she told me that) and in the end, she really was not able to answer the question, "why?" For her, her request for euthanasia was an insurance plan for an unpredictable future and not something that she would choose to do unless reality (and not a distant future) truly became "unbearable."

Other informal rules that impact whether someone's request will go through includes using the right language. Ms. Bosma raised her request appropriately, suggesting it as an option. Others in my sample were not as skillful. For example, you cannot say "I want to die," but you can ask for euthanasia by saying "*Ik wil (het) niet meer*," which means "I don't want it anymore." It is a subtle but distinctive difference to say you do not want to go on anymore versus wishing or wanting death to occur. A wish for death signals possible suicidal thoughts or depression, both red flags for *huisartsen*. Proper euthanasia requests are not death wishes and almost everyone I met who had considered euthanasia did so not because they wanted to die. Most patients I spoke with would have preferred to remain living a healthy life if that were only possible.

There are also rules that include knowing how to behave in proper Dutch ways. Dutch society emphasizes the collective (Horst 2001:19–91), thus when someone who is estranged from family or does not have family involvement requests euthanasia, it raises concerns for the *huisarts*. *Huisartsen* need family to provide an additional perspective and sounding board in the process of euthanasia decision-making. Individuals without family or close friends in The Netherlands (loners and recluses, for example), with the exception of elderly patients who have survived all or most of their living relatives, signal to the *huisarts* that something is wrong. In Ms. Bosma's case, she was not married and had no children, but she was well connected to her father and her sister, both of whom were active participants in her discussions. She also had many friends from her years as a schoolteacher that visited regularly.

Finally, there are characteristics of a patient's case that can result in their exclusion from euthanasia talk. Signs of depression, as I've mentioned, are probably one of the biggest red flags for *huisartsen*. While unbearable suffering for reasons that are psychological in origin are technically acceptable under Dutch law, *huisartsen* would rather not go forward with cases that are based primarily in the realm of psychological suffering. Most *huisartsen* also shy away from cases in which the patient is not terminal or when the disease does not have a predictable trajectory of decline (also allowable under Dutch law). Today, cancer is the disease that is most prevalent in cases of euthanasia, because it is a disease with a somewhat predictable trajectory of decline (unlike, for example, heart disease or multiple conditions that appear in old age). Like Ms. Bosma, 10 of 14 patients in my case study sample had been diagnosed with cancer.[12]

For a number of complex reasons, many foreigners in The Netherlands tend to be excluded from euthanasia discussions. Foreigners who are not citizens are excluded by law[13] and non-native Dutch citizens who are not versed in Dutch manner or do not speak the Dutch language very well tend to be excluded informally. I recall one case in particular, in which a man from Suriname came into the office of his *huisarts* begging to be killed. He was elderly, without any specific illness other than difficulty sleeping and a wish to die. His request was not acknowledged as a request for euthanasia and he was sent home with a new, but limited, prescription for sleeping pills. Many foreigners do not ask for euthanasia and of the ones that did, the most successful foreigners were those who were well versed both in the Dutch language and in Dutch ways of asking for euthanasia. In my sample, there were two patients who were not native Dutch who engaged in euthanasia talk, one was originally from Austria, the other from Germany. Both had lived in The Netherlands many years, married to Dutch natives, and both had learned the language and many of the necessary customs.

---

12. The trends that I found regarding characteristics of euthanasia cases match the trends found in the van der Wal and van der Maas studies. Van der Wal and van der Maas reported in 2001 that 91 percent of all euthanasia cases by *huisartsen* were cases based on diseases of the physical body and that in 77 percent of all euthanasia cases, the main illness reported was cancer (Wal, et al. 2003:47, 49).

13. Foreigners are not allowed under Dutch law to receive euthanasia or assisted suicide. The *Dutch Association for Voluntary End-of-Life (NVVE)* has a form letter they regularly send to foreigners who contact them about euthanasia. This letter states that foreigners cannot receive euthanasia in The Netherlands and should contact resources in their own country. Currently, Switzerland is the only country that accepts foreigners for assisted suicide.

Social Losses and the
Maintenance of Social Bonds

A look at the day-to-day progression of euthanasia talk and the components of euthanasia talk as a discourse begins to expose more complex practices of euthanasia. Euthanasia is clearly not just an end-of-life event; it is a type of discourse that is embedded in cultural and historical practice. While Foucault can help us explain the form and structure of this discourse, we need to explore further to reveal what this discourse means. Thomas Scheff suggests that maintenance of social bonds is the most crucial motive that humans share (Scheff 1990:4). Working from this premise, sociologist Clive Seale (1998) looks at some of the ways that dying disrupts social bonds and what methods people within present-day Anglophone countries are employing in response. Seale writes,

> Disruption of the social bond occurs as the body fails, self-identity becomes harder to hold together and the normal expectations of human relations cannot be fulfilled. In particularly debilitating diseases shame at this failure all too easily surfaces since barriers of privacy may be broken in the invasions of intimacy necessary to maintain a leaking, decaying body, which mirrors a disintegrating sense of self whose boundaries are increasingly beyond control (Seale 1998:149).

Loss of identity disrupts social connections, which can result in *social death*, a death to the social being prior to death of the biological body. According to Seale, social death is a kind of "fall from culture" where individuals can no longer maintain either in language or in bodily form a semblance of sociality. Seale suggests that people resist this fall from culture, however, and they do so in at least two ways: by re-processing loss through therapeutic dialogue to create a more coherent narrative at the end of life or by taking some control over the failing, dying body by manipulating the timing of death to have death of the biological body more closely co-incide with death of the social being.

Narratives at the End of Life. Seale suggests that people employ a kind of socio-therapeutic narrative (what he calls a "revivalist discourse") to stave off social death and maintain a person's sociality. One example he gave was narratives for personal growth that occur as a result of the hospice and palliative care movements in English speaking countries today. By the late 1960s, Elisabeth Kübler-Ross published *On Death and Dying* (1969), a seminal piece that impacted how the dying process was perceived by the public and in medicine. Kübler-Ross was critical of some of the more horrific ways that people were dying due to modernization in medicine. At that time in medical practice, patients were not always told they were dying and Kübler-Ross' book, among others (Glaser and Strauss 1965; Sudnow 1967), argued for full disclosure to patients. Kübler-Ross found dying to be a type of inner journey which if uninterrupted would allow patients and families the time and space they needed to process grief. According to Seale,

> [Kübler-Ross] identifies an initial response of denial, which is then followed by periods of anger, inner bargaining and depression. The final stage of acceptance parallels the adjustment to the reality of loss described in stage models of grief. Both experiences, then, are constructed as a progressive unfolding of inner essence to an eventual resolution, which in the case of dying may be described in beatific or mystical terms (Seale 1998:105).

Seale attributes Kübler-Ross (1969) and others (Glick, et al. 1974; Gorer 1965; Parkes 1972 [1986]) with introducing these stage theories of grief in dying, which provided a cultural script for the good death movement and hospice.

Hospice was founded in the United Kingdom by British nurse and physician Cicley Saunders in the mid 1960s to provide specialized care for the dying. Initially, the focus of hospice was on symptom management and pain control at the end of life. Saunder's concept of pain incorporated physical, emotional, social and spiritual suffering, and families were considered an essential part of the care team (Seale 1998:114–15). According to Seale, hospice is one of the therapeutic narratives that are now available to people who are dying, providing patients and families with a space within the healthcare system to discuss not just physical, but emotional, social and spiritual aspects relevant to end-of-life. Participants in hospice can use these dialogues to construct a sense of meaning that in turn helps maintain sociality for those who are dying.

Euthanasia and Control over the Dying Body. According to Seale, there is another way that people manage social death at the end of life and that is by manipulating the actual timing of biological death—to have death of the body occur generally at the same time as death of the social being. Euthanasia, assisted dying, or refusal of life-sustaining treatments are examples of how people have come to manage social death. Exerting control over the timing and the manner of death allows families the opportunity to avoid the disintegration of the social bond by essentially preempting social death. Seale writes,

> The desire for euthanasia … shares a common root with revivalist discourse in that both are premised on the existence of reflexively aware planning of projects of self-identity, characteristically supported in middle class, Anglophone culture. Both, too, are premised on critiques of modernist medicine. Yet at certain points they diverge, so that support for euthanasia can also be understood as a form of resistance to revivalism (Seale 1998:184).

Seale suggests that a request for euthanasia is the response when a therapeutic narrative alone is not enough to address the damage to social bonds. It can be viewed as demonstrating the limits of cultural constructions or it can be viewed as quite the opposite, as the assertion of culture over nature (Seale 1998:190–91).

Falling from Culture

Dealing with social losses or "falling from culture" are serious concerns at the end of life anywhere and my data suggest that Seale's concept of therapeutic narratives and assertion of control over the body may very well be impacting Dutch end of life. Many of the older patients from my sample of 650 patients included people living with chronic illness and social losses. Losses include incontinence, loss of sight, loss of hearing, inability to drive or do errands, inability to bathe oneself, get out of bed, move independently, inability to eat or feed oneself, onset of dementia and loss of memory (ranging from inability to remember things to inability to recognize loved ones). Not everyone I met experienced the same type or severity of loss, but for those who did lose the ability to participate in one or more daily activities, what they lost was more than simple physical comfort. All of these activities are based a person's ability to participate in their social environment and maintain concepts of identity, relationship and self worth.

Concepts of self and independence seemed to be closely tied to social losses that occurred among the patients and families that I met. There appeared to be a series of milestones that commonly marked loss to self and one's ability to take care of oneself. The term, *onafhankelijk* (independence), was prevalent in the illness narratives I heard and was the term that was used most often to define the social borders of the illness experience. Some of the losses that I heard about most often and in order of their common occurrence were: (1) lost ability to bike and do one's own *boodschappen* (shopping or errands), (2) forced move to institutional care, and (3) incontinence. There were also, however, losses that were not so much talked about as they were demonstrated. The most common of these losses were: (4) social isolation due to death of loved ones, decreasing social circles and an increasingly limited ability to participate in social relationships.

Maintaining Independence. Maintaining independence was how most patients and families framed the illness experience. Losses chipped away at a person's ability to maintain independence and as this occurred, patients and families tended to realign how they defined independence to compensate for one loss after the other. One couple who demonstrated this connection between loss and independence was Mr. and Mrs. Haaring, a couple in their late 80s who were still living at home, but just barely. Their son had died of lung cancer, but they still had an adult daughter and son-in-law who visited once a month and a neighbor who helped them with their *boodschappen* (errands). They received cleaning services twice a week, but had refused to move to the nursing home. When I first met them they were still on the wait list for more extensive home care services. Mr. Haaring was dying. He had been treated for lung cancer and emphysema, and had difficulty eating enough to sustain himself. His wife was also not well and had difficulty getting around. The *huisarts* said if Mr. Haaring did not start eating more, he would die and if anything got worse for either of them he feared they would have to move to a *verpleeghuis* (24 hour care facility). I spoke to Mr. and Mrs. Haaring one day and as they took turns completing each others sentences they told me the story of how they ran a fruit and vegetable store for many years and how they loved to travel. Now, they told me, Mr. Haaring cannot work, he cannot do his *boodschappen,* he got hit by a flying umbrella on the Italian shore last year and they are not sure if he is well enough to return. He used to swim but cannot do that anymore. I asked if he can walk and he says yes, to the bathroom. They want to go back to Italy where elders are treated very well by their children. In Italy they tell me elders live with their children. Do you want to live with your children, I ask? No they tell me, because they are *onafhanke-lijk* (independent).

Biking and Boodschappen *(Errands).* One of the most common losses in The Netherlands and typically the first milestone of social loss that occurs are the related abilities to bike and do one's own *boodschappen* (errands). The Netherlands is an incredible country for biking. The entire country is connected by bike paths, much like the U.S. is connected by our highway system. Bikers have their own lanes (separated from both car and foot traffic) with stoplights to regulate the flow with other traffic. Virtually everyone in The Netherlands rides a bike. Physicians allow infants in bike seats as soon as they are able to sit up on their own; older children ride their own bike next to an adult who rides with a hand on the child's shoulder for protection; adults ride bikes everywhere; and persons who are elderly will continue to ride as long as possible, substituting their bicycle for a motorized scooter when balance and safety become a concern. Biking in The Netherlands is part of what it is to live and move in Dutch ways. I remember a scene from a Steve Martin movie, *LA Stories*, where one of the characters, living in Los Angeles, jumps in the car to drive to a location one block away, implying with some humor that people in Los Angeles drive everywhere they go. It is like that in The Netherlands, but with bicycles instead of cars. Dutch people bike everywhere—to work, to go out at night, on errands, and for pleasure.

Biking, *boodschappen* and concepts of independence are closely linked and so it is not surprising that it was one of the most talked about milestones of social loss among the Dutch families I met. Each neighborhood has its own collection of shops: the butcher, the flower shop, the bread shop, the sweet shop, the vegetable stand, the cheese shop, and if you still needed something, the all-inclusive grocery store. On the weekends, open-air markets sold a variety of food, flowers, and inexpensive household and clothing items. Shopping for fresh food and flowers and going to the various shops that have the best products for the best price is something Dutch people do regularly, riding through the streets with their bagged purchases balanced on each side of the steering wheel or in packs off the back wheel. Many whom I met when asked about their illness included in their response a clarification that they either could or could no longer do their own *boodschappen*. One woman I met was in her 80s living in a *bejaardenhuis* (a nursing home for persons who are elderly). She had slight dementia and walked with a very slow shuffle aided by a rolling walker, but what she lacked physically she made up for in personality. She explained to her doctor that she had been thinking about getting one of those motorized bicycles so that she could get out and around again. She thought it best that she check with him before buying this. Clearly, she was no longer capable of biking and her doctor told her this was not a good idea. But she pressed on, suggesting that maybe she really should get this bike and reiterating that she's been thinking about it. Her doctor again said no and asked if he should call her daughter to let her know his decision.

Move to Institutional Care. The move from home to a facility was another common milestone of social loss. While many elderly in The Netherlands have the opportunity to stay at home to die through an extensive system of social medicine, public welfare and homecare, the numbers of persons who die in institutional care still outnumber home deaths. In The Netherlands in 2003, approximately one third of all deaths were in the hospital, more than one quarter were at home and one fifth of all deaths were in nursing or acute care homes (CBS 2004). Institutional care in The Netherlands includes hospitals (*ziekenhuizen*), nursing homes (*verzorgingscentra*) and acute care facilities (*verpleeghuizen*). Nursing homes and acute care facilities are institutions that provide 24-hour nursing care and assistance and are typically viewed as providing the highest level of care outside of a hospital setting. Also available are independent or assisted living (*aanleunwoning*) and homes for the elderly (*bejaardenhuizen*), institutions that provide limited assistance with nursing and daily living care and typically viewed as providing lower levels of care. In The Netherlands, approximately 9.0 percent of persons 65 or older live in nursing homes or residential homes compared to 6.5 percent in the U.S. (Ribbe 2004). We know that in both countries the trend over the last century was toward institutional care at the end of life, but in the last few decades the trend has reversed as more people in both countries are staying in the home longer and using more outpatient services (CBS 2004; CBS 2008a; IOM 1997; Pandya 2001).

Most Dutch people move to a facility when there is no longer a choice to stay at home, and once they move many I met adjusted fairly well to their new life. Mr. van Sluit was 87 when he moved to a residential home (*aanleuning*). His wife had suffered from dementia and he cared for her at home as long as he could, until his leg was amputated due to complications from diabetes. He moved to the *aanleuning* (independent living) section of the *bejaardenhuis* (elder care home) when he couldn't live by himself anymore. His wife died not soon after. I asked him how it was to move and he said,

> *Ja.* First it was difficult, naturally. When you live 60 years in your own house together and then [one day] you can't do anything, you're laid up. Everything was gone and I didn't feel at home here. But *ik woon mooi, ik heb een mooi uitzicht* (I live well; I have a good outlook [on life]). I have my own room, my own furniture that I brought with me, and that gives you a *vertrouwd* (familiar or trustworthy) feeling because my kids live close by, my two daughters, they come and visit regularly. Through that I have a lot of support and that makes life *prettig* (pleasant or nice).

Mr. van Sluit's reaction to moving was similar to many I met. For those who were still living at home, they clearly did not want to move to an institution, but once they did many found a way to come to terms with it. Part of the adjustment to institutional care is eased by the interior setting of Dutch facilities, which are styled to look more like homes than U.S. nursing facilities typically are.[14] In The Netherlands, people are encouraged to bring their own furniture and decorations from home and often the only piece of institutional furniture in a room might be the hospital bed. Coffee and tea breaks are a social affair, held at regularly scheduled times in the break room, which like the other rooms is decorated similar to a Dutch living room.

---

14. The appearance of nursing and acute care facilities are beginning to change in the U.S. Assisted living centers, such as Sunrise Living modeled after the Dutch system of care, are in stark contrast to the white walls and linoleum floors of the more traditional nursing home in the U.S. The shift is from a more hospital-like interior towards a more home-like setting. For more on alternatives to traditional nursing homes in the U.S., see (Gleckman 2009).

Others did not adjust as well because after all, it was what it was—a substitute home when family support was no longer available or not enough to handle complications at the end of life. Even Mr. van Sluit had his low days, which I'm certain were compounded by the death of his wife and his increasingly limited circumstances.

Incontinence. Probably one of the more difficult losses, one that I saw the most tears over, was incontinence or the inability to control the flow of urine (and in some cases, fecal matter). One day an elderly couple in their 70s came into the doctor's office. The man had recently returned home from an operation to remove bowel cancer and immediately he starts to cry, head in hands. He just had the catheter out yesterday and now he is peeing in the bed, he has no control over it, and he wakes up wet and cold. Dr. Muller lets him talk for a while then asks softly, "What will make you feel better? Staying in bed?" "I have no control," the man says crying again, "In bed I feel *gelukkig* (well and happy), out of bed I can't even control when I'm going to pee. I can't even feel it." Dr. Muller asks what drugs he is taking and his wife starts to list them. The *huisarts* listens then offers some solutions, which the man seems to like. Dr. Muller asks if there is any other problem today. But the woman says no and the man talks about the wetness again. "My brother died from bowel cancer and he has kids and grandkids," he says. Dr. Muller suggests he may be feeling depressed and it is important to get out of bed and do things when he feels like that. We will consult with the urologist, he says, and see if we can fix the peeing problem first.

There was something about incontinence that really struck a chord not only with this man, but also with many of the people I met who shared this problem. Incontinence typically brought some of the most heart-wrenching tears from patients. For the man in this excerpt, he connected incontinence as a step towards death, just like his brother who died of bowel cancer. But there was also something just about that step from being able to control one's body to losing control that left an imprint. Mary Douglas offers an enlightening look at the transgression of bodily boundaries in her book, *Purity and Danger* (1966). In it, she suggests that the orifices of the body and the matter that issues forth, such as urine or feces, symbolize the body's most dangerous and vulnerable points. According to Douglas, dirt is decay is death, but to understand the symbolic role of death in ritual, one must better understand when dirt, typically something treated as taboo, becomes something creative, something constructive to society. Dirt reveals the boundaries, the "vulnerable margins," of society and no margin is more vulnerable than the orifices of the body. Douglas explains,

> Any structure of ideas is vulnerable at its margins. We should expect the orifices of the body to symbolise its specially vulnerable points. Matter issuing from them is marginal stuff of the most obvious kind. Spittle, blood, milk, urine, faeces or tears by simply issuing forth have traversed the boundary of the body (Douglas 1966:122).

My time spent with people who are dying revealed that dying is often a messy business. At the end, many sick rooms have a distinctive odor of the fluids the body can no longer contain and that efforts to clean can no longer mask. For some there are wounds that do not heal, skin and tissue that rots on the body, and tumors that drain pus and blood. Catheters channel urine to bags hanging bedside and the smell of vomit or feces hangs in the air. Many suffer urinary incontinence and for some it signaled a first step towards losing control over the body.

Loneliness and Social Isolation. One of the more subtle, but powerful, social losses that I saw among the patients I met was the loss of relationships and the resulting loneliness and social isolation that occurs when people near the end of life. As one woman I visited put it, everyone else she knew was dead. Ms. Rozemond was 91 years old living in a nursing home (*verzorgingscentrum*). She had been a teacher for many years then met a woman pianist with whom she became very connected. Over time her pianist friend died, her parents died and each of her siblings died. She says she has no *doel* (purpose, goal) in life anymore. No one needs her anymore and she's not able to get around anymore. I ask if she has friends in the nursing home and Mrs. Rozemond replies, "Not really friends. I have acquaintances. Coffee time is at 10:00 a.m. here and usually I go for that but when I do go they sit there and don't speak. People here have a bit of dementia, but "*mijn koppie is nog steeds goed* (my head is still good)," she says pointing to her head.

Social isolation does not occur in quite the same way in The Netherlands as it does in the U.S. Just as in the U.S., women in The Netherlands tend to outlive males and many of my visits, particularly in institutional care, were with women who had been widowed. While very few invoked the word for loneliness, *eenzaamheid*, I heard and saw complaints of not feeling useful anymore, of having little left to do, and of dwindling relationships as friends and family died and left them alone. But isolation and loneliness in The Netherlands stand in contradiction to a society that is based in the collective. Dutch people are encouraged to be together, but to "*doe maar gewoon dat is gek genoeg* (be normal that is crazy enough)." In other words, they are encouraged not to isolate themselves in relationships or by rising above or standing out from the collective. The fact is that the Dutch spend much of their time together.

As a single person living in Amsterdam, I quickly felt this emphasis on the collective. I lived with a family in Utrecht for a month and found that retiring to my room for privacy after dinner and an hour or so of conversation was still too early. Family spends its time together, even if that means reading your book in the corner of the living room. In restaurants, I noticed acutely how single diners are often placed at a large, long table so that they do not technically dine alone. Frequently in response to work stress or stress in a marriage or slight depression, I heard *huisartsen* suggest that patients get out, go biking or join one of the many social, sporting, or hobby-based clubs. Loners are not the norm in Dutch society.

So why then do elderly couples like the Haarings prefer to move into institutional care rather than into homes with adult children when they can no longer stay at home themselves? Social historian Han van der Horst suggests that while Dutch elderly may be lonely, their desire for independence and self-sufficiency take precedence. He writes,

> [the] average life expectancy [for Dutch women] is 78 and, as in most countries, they tend to outlive their husbands. Behind their impeccable white net curtains, they endure their unhappiness in silence, because they find it difficult to express their emotions. They put on a brave face and hide their misery from outsiders. This is due partly to pride, partly to embarrassment and partly because they don't want to be a nuisance. The obvious thing to do is to bring these lonely people together, and many attempts are made. They are, however, rarely successful because the loneliness is often partly founded on the desire to be left to one's own devices and not be dependent on anyone (Horst 2001:230).

In The Netherlands, being an independent, yet socially connected and useful member of society is core.

Assertions of Control: A Look at Dutch Responses to Social Loss and Social Death

I have talked about how euthanasia is most often experienced as a discussion rather than a life-ending act and with the aid of Foucault, I have been able to delineate some of the elements that make up this end-of-life discourse. I have also talked a little about the context of dying in The Netherlands, a context based in longer periods of decline and inevitable social losses. The question remains, however, what is the Dutch response to social loss and, ultimately, social death? Do Dutch people maintain sociality at the end of life by therapeutic narratives and practices that realign the timing of social and biological death?

My data suggests the answer is yes and no. Consider Ms. Bosma's story. Hers was typical of the euthanasia discussions that I saw take place. All of these discussions are orchestrated by the *huisarts;* family members are always encouraged (and frankly expected) to participate; and discussions typically speak not only to simply the matter at hand (planning a euthanasia death), but also are orchestrated to elicit how the patient and the family are feeling and what the meaning of death and loss has for them. Ironically, the practice that is ostensibly for the purpose of planning death becomes a practice for reaffirming life, sociality and the roles that Dutch people assume even in the face of social losses and impending death. Through this process sociality is re-worked and concepts of identity solidified.

Euthanasia talk is a kind of therapeutic narrative, based on a tendency to reassert order and coherence after the onslaught of social loss, the disruption of concepts of self, and one's ability to participate in social life. Medical anthropologist, Gay Becker (1997) suggests that body and the voice that narrates our own experience of the body are intimately connected. When disruption occurs, such as loss of mobility or incontinence, the body becomes something unfamiliar and unbalanced. The human tendency is to restore continuity, to re-work how the disruption is viewed and understood. In our case of the man with incontinence, for example, that would be him re-writing his own narrative from something like 'incontinence is the first step towards death' to 'many people suffer from incontinence and so do I.' Transformative narratives are employed to repair and re-order breaks in concepts of self and other.

As for assertions of control over the body, I think that is in large part what is occurring *both in language and in practice.* Assertions over the manner and timing of death are not simply played out in the physical realm where patients follow-through with requests for euthanasia, assisted suicide or other medical behaviors that potentially shorten life. Assertions of control are also played out on symbolic and emotional levels, where euthanasia talk provides participants with the language and the social space for re-working end of life experience. Participants can use a future ideal of a peaceful euthanasia death to make the present reality of social loss less debilitating.

CHAPTER 3

EUTHANASIA IN HISTORICAL
AND CULTURAL PERSPECTIVE

April 10th, 2001 was a crisp, sunny day in The Hague, the kind of day that we visitors to Holland look forward to after a long, wet winter with only rare glimpses of the sun. It was the same day that a bill legalizing euthanasia was debated and passed by the First Chamber of the Dutch legislature, solidifying The Netherlands as the country with the longest-standing, legal practice of euthanasia. I arrived in The Hague by train and met my colleague and friend, Albert Klijn, a socio-legal researcher with the Ministry of Justice (WODC). It was 10 o'clock in the morning and by 10 o'clock that night members of the First Chamber were expected to vote on whether or not to pass the Termination of Life on Request and Assisted Suicide (Review Procedures) Act. *It was a symbolic gesture by a liberal majority made up of the Labor Party (PvdA), the People's Party for Freedom and Democracy (VVD), and Democrats '66 (D66). The "Purple Cabinet" as they were popularly called, together with the Green Party (GL), would move the much-debated practice of euthanasia legalized by court decision in 1984 into the realm of legislation.*

Albert and I find the public viewing room located one building over from the First Chamber. This is where people without tickets can sit and view history being made by satellite feed. There are surprisingly few people here. Outside, only a handful of protestors—one group of four standing around a van with the back doors opened to reveal a large statue of the Virgin Mary and another group of about 20 assembled around a priest in robes. The priest was speaking quietly to the crowd. Both groups are decidedly tame, even by Dutch standards.

Inside, the viewing room is stark with a line of mostly empty folding chairs facing a large television screen. Maybe 20 to 30 people are scattered around the room.

Albert fills me in. He says the Chamber convened last night at 7:00 p.m. with opening statements by the spokespersons of each political party. The Termination of Life on Request and Assisted Suicide (Review Procedures) Act, *as it is called, passed the Second Chamber in November 2000 and with the current liberal coalition in place, Albert says, there is no question that the law will pass the First Chamber today.*[1] *I've read something about the Dutch system. It is an interesting one based on a multiple party system that regularly sees as many as 12 or more parties winning seats in both the First (Upper) and Second (Lower) Chambers. This means that no one party wins a majority, but there are a few who tend to come out on top. Once elections are completed, those with the most seats and similar politics will band together to form a coalition. In 2001, PvdA, VVD, D66, and the Green Party formed the majority coalition supporting the euthanasia law, which was opposed most vocally by the Christian Democrat Party (CDA), the Socialist Party (SP), and three small orthodox Calvinist parties.*[2] *According to Albert, the liberal majority formed out of the elections of 1994, taking over the majority position from a more conservative Christian-right coalition. The Purple Cabinet, he thought,*

---

1. The Dutch Parliament, like ours, is made up of two houses: the First Chamber (equivalent to our Senate) and the Second Chamber (equivalent to our House of Representatives). Legislation must begin in the Second Chamber where members have the ability to amend proposals and then must be either accepted or rejected by the First Chamber.

2. The majority parties in opposition over the proposed euthanasia law were as follows. The majority in favor of the law were PvdA (the labor party), VVD (known as the traditional liberal party), D66 (liberals thought to be left of VVD), and GL (the swing party made up of the former Communist Party, environmentalists and former Catholic politicians). Parties opposing the law included CDA (the Christian Democrats), SP (the left-leaning socialist party), SGP, RPF and GPV (three orthodox Calvinist parties, represented by one speaker in the debates, Mr. Schuurman).

saw their time in office as a "window of opportunity" to turn away from more conservative, religious right policies and to pass, instead, policies that support what they believed were popularly held beliefs around social life in The Netherlands. Since their election, the Purple Cabinet have passed laws supporting same sex partnerships, marriages and, on today's agenda—euthanasia.

This morning it is time for the Ministers of Justice (Korthals) and Health, Welfare and Sport (Borst) to speak, to reply to comments made last night by Chamber members. First the Ministers will speak; Chamber members can reply; the Ministers will speak again; and then the members will vote. We watch the television screen and Albert tells me that the First Chamber is known as a "chamber of reflection." Members must vote yes or no, but they cannot make amendments or changes to the bill. They can, however, offer suggestions and hope that their suggestions get incorporated. Unlike the Second Chamber, the First is arranged so that all party members are seated mixed throughout the room, instead of allowing party affiliates to sit together. This, he thinks, facilitates the "reflection" aspect.

I focus on the screen and hear Timmerman-Buck (CDA) ask about the reporting procedure for physicians performing euthanasia. She asks what happens when we normalize euthanasia, as opposed to having euthanasia be an exception to the law. Minister Korthals talks about reporting frequencies (how often doctors are reporting euthanasia) and mentions the van der Wal and van der Maas studies (originally called the Remmelink Study, commissioned by the government to study the prevalence of euthanasia and other related practices). Timmerman-Buck pushes, saying we want more doctors to report when they are performing euthanasia; that is the goal of the euthanasia law, right? Minister Korthals agrees and says they will prosecute doctors if they fail to report.

Next, Minister Borst begins her speech. She says that the proposed law reflects a "respect for life" and she reminds us that the world is watching. In our system, she says, you can have care until the "bitter end" and mentions the role of nurses who give patients the time and space to talk about what they want at the end of their life. Schuurman (RPF/GPV) interrupts Borst. He says he is worried that euthanasia will become an obligation. There are shortages in available care, which might make euthanasia too easy an option. Minister Borst counters, saying "a euthanasia request is not euthanasia" and that "no one is obliged to ask for euthanasia." Schuurman interrupts again to talk about the "toetsingscommissies," *the regional review committees set up in 1998 to monitor the Requirements of Due Care as outlined by the Royal Dutch Medical Association. Are they doing their job, Schuurman asks. Minister Borst continues, reflecting on the importance of palliative care. "Good palliative care," she says, "is integral to good healthcare."*

I ask Albert, what's up with all the interruptions? He tells me that that is how it works. Members can interrupt the Minister's speech at any time, with no acknowledgement from the chairman (the moderator) or the speaker. Members must only walk up to the podium and speak into the microphone. Borst and Chamber members continue the dance, "reflecting" on the role of the regional review committees, the role of the doctors, nurses, religion and government.

We break for lunch and Albert scores two passes for us to sit in the chamber for the remainder of the day. At one o'clock the First Chamber reconvenes to talk briefly about the Constantijn marriage (they are voting on whether to approve the marriage of the Queen's son), with plans to continue with euthanasia discussions at 3:30 p.m. We enter the First Chamber by the second floor balcony, where visitors are allowed to sit to view the proceedings below. It is a magnificent room befitting such an occasion. It is a large hall arranged similarly to a Dutch church where the members face each other, rather than facing a central altar. Small, two-seater pews are arranged in rows and members face each other at a slight angle. The visitor balconies are similarly situated, located on opposite sides of the room, so that visitors can observe each other and the events below. At the top of the room is the chairman's table and at the bottom, the Minister's table. The four sides are arranged like a trapezoid, with everyone facing inward. The chairman is dwarfed by a large painting of King Willem II, the second king of an independent Netherlands who swore in the first parliamentary cabinet before his death in 1848 (Schama 1987:65; Shetter 1987:226). The ceiling, too, speaks in history, covered by murals depicting a building with windows and people from various cultures looking in. I see what appears to be Dutch people in the dress of the 17th century, Indonesians and Africans, and interspersed throughout cherubs supporting the frames of the building, all observing the proceedings from their place on high. Below this, the wall is lined with portraits of elderly, white Dutch men, probably original chamber members is my guess. Albert tells me the building is a new building, which they decided to keep in the "old style."

The euthanasia debates get started again and Timmerman-Buck from CDA is running through all the elements of current euthanasia practice that may throw the law into question: What about passive euthanasia? What is the role of the regional review committees? How can we say that reporting will increase under the new law? And what about dementia and euthanasia? Kohnstam from D66 says there is a history to euthanasia, but that voluntary euthanasia "has totally nothing to do with Nazi Germany." He disagrees with Schuurman and Timmerman-Buck. Schuurman says he feels misunderstood, says there is a break in society and reads a passage (in English) about dying with dignity. Chamber members, I note, are starting to look bored. Several look like they are sleeping off lunch, propping their heads politely off their tables using hands and elbows. Schuurman makes a motion asking for more support and training for palliative care. The chairman reads the motion then asks for comments for and against. De Wolff from the Green Party says euthanasia will not be normalized by this law and cites a recent newspaper article by a foreigner who said that the Dutch have figured out their moral society. She agrees and will favor this law today. Le Poole from the Labor Party (PvdA) says that doctors stuck their neck out for this policy and this is for them and their patients who have thought about what they want. She too mentions Nazi Germany and outsider reactions. Dees from VVD starts to quote an English text regarding right to choice and is interrupted, reminded that the text was not originally in English, therefore he should paraphrase it in Dutch. Ruers from the Socialist Party (SP) wonders who is controlling the regional review (toetsing) committees. Nobody, he says.

I lean in closer to Albert to ask how many will speak on this motion and he tells me seven — seven parties, seven spokespersons. The remaining chamber members speak, then the chairman reminds speakers about the rules for using other languages in the chamber. If a text is available in Dutch, even if it has been translated from another language, members must use the Dutch version. The chamber breaks for an hour, with plans to reconvene at 6:00 p.m. Outside there are only a few news cameras and one new set of protestors: two men in black ski masks and white lab coats with over-sized syringes in their pockets and a larger banner that reads "Euthanasie blijft moord, 293 294 WvSr," which translates to "Euthanasia is still murder" and cites the main articles of the criminal code that will be altered by the passage of the law today. Below the inscription is the familiar red circle with a slash through the Dutch words for "constitutional state" and "civilization." Over beers at a local pub, I ask about the protestors and the media. Where are they? I ask. Albert says it is a done deal so most of the protestors stayed home and much of the media presence are probably foreign. It was not until the next day that I found out that a crowd of protestors did gather to stage a rally, but they did it in a courtyard across the street and out of sight of the First Chamber building at the request of officials. A polite Dutch protest I think to myself.

The chamber reconvenes at 6:00 p.m. The chairman calls the room to order and Minister Korthals begins reading from some typed notes. He is responding to Timmerman's position on the regional review committees. Timmerman-Buck interrupts. She is starting to get emotional. Minister Borst reads from her typed notes on palliative care. She says palliative care is not separate from other care at the end of life in the sense that it is all offered through Thuiszorg *(the government-subsidized, national homecare organization). Borst thinks Schuurman's motion is unnecessary. Schuurman says he wants to keep his motion. The chairman suggests a 20-minute break so that CDA and their coalition can meet. The chamber reconvenes at 7:20 and I note that the mood in the chamber has shifted somewhat. The seats on the chamber floor are full, the balcony is overflowing and the mood is one of excitement. I assume we are getting close to a vote. Albert points out some of the members of the Second Chamber who have joined us on the balcony to watch. We are all leaning forward in our seats now. The chairman says we will take a vote on the motion and asks if someone wants to speak. Timmerman-Buck steps up to do so, saying only a few brief words. Turn by turn, one member from each party gets up to speak to the motion. They are all brief. Next, the chairman calls for a vote on the euthanasia bill, members must say for or against when their name is called. He begins calling names. Albert tells me that only a simple majority is needed to pass (38 of 75 members "for" will pass the bill). The vote comes in — it is 46 for, 28 against, and 1 not present. The bill passes in silence; no clapping, no noise. Next there is a vote on the motion and members are asked to stand to vote for it. The motion fails and then everyone is up out of their seats, shaking hands and congratulating their neighbors. I, too, receive handshakes and congratulations. On the floor of the chamber I see one young member, who I didn't hear from all day, put his head on his desk. He appears to be crying. Several members join him, one leaning in to offer words of comfort and a hand on the back.*

On April 10, 2001, the Dutch parliament approved the *Termination of Life on Request and Assisted Suicide (Review Procedures) Act* making the 1984 court-sanctioned practice of euthanasia (killing a person at that person's explicit request) and assisted suicide (giving a person the means to kill themselves at that person's explicit request) legal by statute in The Netherlands.[3] After 30 some years of national debate and 17 years of legal practice, The Netherlands became the country with the longest-standing legal practice of euthanasia and assisted suicide in the world.

---

3. The Dutch distinguish between euthanasia and assisted suicide. Euthanasia occurs more often than assisted suicide for reasons that include a general trust in physicians, a long-standing policy of social medicine, and the belief that euthanasia is safer (quicker and more dependable) than assisted suicide. In 2001, approximately 2.6 percent of all deaths were attributed to euthanasia, while only 0.2 percent of all deaths were attributed to assisted suicide (Wal, et al. 2003:46).

The Parliamentary debates on April 10, 2001 tell us a story that is enmeshed in a Dutch way of being. We, the reader, arrive in the middle of the story to find that euthanasia law in The Netherlands is a done deal. It seems a symbolic gesture capping years of mainstream practice. We meet the political players — proponents of the law (Ministers Borst and Korthals, and spokespersons from VVD, D66, PvdA, and GL) and opponents of the law (CDA, RFP, SGP, GPV, and SP) and we hear briefly of some of the most pressing concerns: whether Dutch doctors are regularly reporting euthanasia cases, whether regional review (*toetsing*) committees are capable of regulating lawful practice, and whether Dutch standards of palliative care are sufficient.

This is not just a Dutch story, however, because as Minister Borst and other Dutch leaders reminded us that day, "the world is watching." Foucault's concept of discourse suggests that Dutch practices and policies at the end of life are influenced both by elements of which Dutch participants are aware and by elements of which participants may not be aware. In this chapter I will explore both key historical events and those underlying elements of history and culture that appear to be impacting end-of-life discourse in The Netherlands and in the U.S. So many have written entire books about the history of euthanasia and other related practices, thus my goal here is not to condense what has been done more thoroughly elsewhere but instead to highlight just those aspects in history and culture that I see as impacting end-of-life practices and policies in The Netherlands and in the U.S.[4]

---

4. There have been many books written about the history of euthanasia and other related practices. The most accurate and detailed account of the Dutch legal experience can be found in two books by Griffiths et al. (Griffiths, et al. 1998; Griffiths, et al. 2008). For a good discussion of the pros and cons of euthanasia world-wide, see (Foley and Hendin 2002; Quill and Battin 2004). Dowbiggin offers a detailed history of euthanasia from a con-perspective (Dowbiggin 2005). James Kennedy offers a thoughtful social-historical review of the Dutch experience in the Dutch language (Kennedy 2002; Kennedy 1995) and Shai Lavi offers a thoughtful socio-

Connection to Suicide

The story begins with the connection that modern-day euthanasia and assistance in dying continue to share with suicide. Emile Durkheim (1951) was one of the early social scientists to conduct a full-length study of suicide. He argued that suicide should not be attributed to factors that are psychological or environmental, such as the impact of cold weather climates. He argued that the cause of suicide is social, based in flaws in the social integration of the person with his or her society. Durkheim identified three forms of suicide: *egoistic*, resulting from a lack of integration of an individual with society; *altruistic*, resulting from over-integration of an individual with society; and *anomic*, in which social regulations are not functioning properly (Durkheim 1951:145–276).

Could euthanasia be a modern-day form of altruistic suicide? It is a compelling argument that suggests that perhaps Dutch people are over-integrated with their own society, offering themselves for early death because state policy and public discourses may be subtly pushing citizens towards euthanasia as a response to terminal prognosis. Perhaps euthanasia is a form of anomic suicide in the sense that by opening legal euthanasia for those who really may need it, it paves the way for non-legal suicides. Persons simply wishing to die may learn how to "work the system" to disguise their suicide as legally-supported euthanasia or doctors may be disguising suicide or homicide in other medical practices that hasten death, such as terminal sedation or withholding or withdrawal of support.

In practice, surprisingly, euthanasia and assisted suicide in The Netherlands are not a wish for death. The people I met did not want to die. What people did at the end of life, however, was draw

---

historical perspective of the American experience in the English language (Lavi 2005).

lines in the sand. Someone would say, "I don't want to go on if I cannot do my art anymore" or "I will want euthanasia once they remove my other leg," but invariably as that line in the sand approached, many incorporated their new limitation only to draw another line in the sand for another day. As you will see when you read Part II of this book, euthanasia talk for the majority of participants is more about an insurance policy for future suffering and euthanasia death is the choice typically when all avenues of sociality have been exhausted.

As concepts, however, euthanasia and assisted dying remain bound with historical events and moral arguments around suicide. In history, euthanasia and assisted dying have often been viewed as two of the more accepted forms of suicide, typically for reasons of illness, infirmity or old age (Lam 1997). In Antiquity, Greeks and Romans took any number of stances toward suicide, including the popular thought that suicide was a rational choice of free men. Any number of famous and not so famous ancient Greeks and Romans took their own lives, including Pythagoras, Diogenes, Zeno, Socrates, Cato, Epicurus, Seneca and tens of thousands of Christian martyrs who offered themselves for public annihilation in Roman coliseums for the promise of salvation in the Hereafter. Greek Epicureans promoted suicide as a rational choice when life became intolerable. The Stoics also recommended suicide as a rational choice. According to Diogenes Laertius, "the wise man can with reason give his life for his country and his friends, or he can kill himself if he suffers serious pain, if he has lost a limb, or if he has an incurable illness" (quoted in Minois 1999:42–4).

It was not until the Christian era that suicide entered the realm of taboo, namely as a sin against God. The early years of Christianity were marked by ambivalence toward suicide, but under the influence of St. Augustine, the Church came to adopt a more cohesive stance against suicide. Following on Plato's argument in *Phaedo* and in reaction to Donatists who defended Christian martyrdom, St. Augustine based his argument on the Sixth Commandment, "thou shall not kill." In *City of God,* St. Augustine argues that no man has the right to end his life, no matter the motivation.

St. Augustine argued that man is created in His image and life is the gift of God, thus a rejection of life is a rejection of God (Alvarez 1971:50; Minois 1999:27–28). By mid century, Christian law followed suit with a series of prohibitions, solidifying the Church's stance against all forms of suicide. In 452, the Council of Arles, forbade suicide of slaves and domestic servants and in 533 the Council of Orléans forbade suicide of accused criminals. In 563 and 578, the Councils of Braga and Auxerre, respectively, forbade all forms of suicide, making it an offense against God which resulted in damnation in the hereafter and punishment both in terms of the suicide's possessions and remains (Minois 1999:29–30).

Today, assisted dying has once again emerged in the public domain as one of the more accepted forms of suicide. While it is a practice that has continued to occur throughout history, it has most recently come to the attention of the public as a medical and legal concern. Advocates have attempted to legitimize the practice by distancing assisted dying for reasons of terminal or incurable illness from historical connections with suicide and the taboos that have surrounded suicide. As medical science emerged as a discipline in the 19th and 20th centuries, death became increasingly a medical concern. Physicians and medicine began to replace chaplains and religion at the bedside of the sick and the dying. Key advances in medicine, such as the advent of antisepsis techniques in surgery and most recently the ability to maintain oxygen flow via the artificial ventilator, allowed many people to live longer lives, but they also meant that suffering was prolonged (Lynn 2004:4–31). This led to important ethical questions in public debates around the world about what constitutes quality of life, particularly at the end of life (Lock 2002:57–75; Starr 1982:145–162).

There are only a few countries in which euthanasia or assisted dying (sometimes called "voluntary and active euthanasia")[5] are legally

---

5. Outside of The Netherlands, euthanasia has been categorized as active-passive or voluntary-involuntary. Active euthanasia includes practices where steps are taken to induce death, such as injecting or ingesting a lethal dose of medication, whereas passive euthanasia is withdrawing or

practiced, but many more places where it regularly occurs. I use the term, *legal practice*, to denote both formal legal acceptance (by judicial decision or by legislation) and common occurrence. Today, euthanasia is legally practiced in The Netherlands (since 1984) and Belgium (since 2002). Physician-assisted dying is legally practiced in The Netherlands (since 1984), in Belgium (since 2002), in Switzerland (since 1937), and in the state of Oregon in the United States (since 1997). Euthanasia is technically legal in Colombia (since 1997) and physician-assisted dying is technically legal in Germany (since 1751), but in both places regular and open practices have not been established. In Japan, where they have a long history of suicide for reasons of honor (*hara-kiri*, *seppuku*, and *Kamikaze* pilots), euthanasia is technically legal (since 1962), but is typically associated with the withdrawal or withholding of support and not ending a person's life by lethal injection. Euthanasia was legal for a brief period in Australia (1996–1997) only to be overturned. In 2008, voters in the state of Washington joined Oregon by passing Initiative 1000, legalizing physician-assisted dying in the second U.S. state. In 2009, Luxembourg became the third EU country to legalize euthanasia and assisted suicide (AFP 2008; Goldstein 2008; Heide, et al. 2003; SCBI 2002; Scherer and Simon 1999).

We also know that forms of euthanasia and assisted suicide regularly occur in countries where it is not legal. We have testimonial accounts from family and friends (Humphry 1978; Keizer 1996; Rollin 1987; Shavelson 1995) and from physician surveys that suggest that practices similar to euthanasia and physician-assisted dying are occurring around the world, including in Europe, Australia, Japan, and the United States (Emanuel, et al. 2000; Heide, et al. 2003; Magnusson 2004; Meier, et al. 1998; Morita, et al. 2002).

---

withholding life-sustaining treatments or medications. Both practices can either be categorized as voluntary (at the patient's explicit request or consent) or involuntary (not at the patient's explicit request or consent).

Euthanasia and Assisted Dying in Historical Perspective

The historical development of the Dutch stance toward euthanasia and assisted suicide can be distinguished from the American perspective by two important factors. First, the Dutch debate has largely been a physician-led movement which began when physicians in The Netherlands voiced their frustration with technologies at the end of life that were allowing patients to live longer but at a cost to quality of life. Unlike in the U.S. where the movement is predominantly framed as a patient's right against physicians and the medical system to determine end-of-life, in The Netherlands the doctor-patient relationship is not so contentious. Second, as a result the focus in The Netherlands has been on euthanasia, allowing the physician to end life typically by lethal injection, whereas in the U.S. the debates have focused around assisted dying, where patients take the initiative to end their own lives typically with prescription drugs prescribed but not administered by the physician. Fundamentally, these historical developments have created two very different perspectives on end of life. The following details some of the main historical events that have led to current day assisted dying policy and practices in The Netherlands and in the U.S.

The Dutch Experience

Distancing from Hitler's "Euthanasia" Program. By the 1930s and '40s, euthanasia had been on the European radar for some time, marked by a decrease in church membership and in Germany by the pivotal work, *Die Freigabe der Vernichtung Lebensunweren Lebens* (The Permission to Destroy Life Unworthy of Life). Written by German jurist, Karl Binding, and professor of psychiatry, Alfred Hoche (1920) this work provided the rationale for killing disabled infants, adults and persons who were terminally ill, and paved the way for the Nazi-led Holocaust. In this text, Binding and Hoche stressed the therapeutic nature of euthanasia and argued that only doctors should be legally responsible for assisting in death for those deemed "unworthy of life" (Lifton 1986:45–50). In July 1933, Hitler came out with his Law for the Prevention of Progeny with Hereditary Diseases, legalizing involuntary sterilization and abortion of fetuses. In 1939, Hitler instituted the *Aktion T4* Program—a "euthanasia" program that included adults with chronic disabilities, incurable illnesses, and persons not of German descent. The T4 program was expanded under Hitler's regime and by 1941 was attributed with the deaths of an estimated 75,000 to 250,000 men, women and children.

The war began with the invasion of Austria in 1938 and between 1938 and 1945, the Germans opened numerous concentration camps, forced-labor and extermination camps for those deemed unworthy of life. By the end of the war, it is estimated that as many as 6 million men, women and children (most of them Jewish) were killed under the auspices of "euthanasia" and racial cleansing. News of the killings began to trickle out of Nazi occupied areas, but came to light most clearly during the Nuremberg trials with Nazi physicians in 1946 and 1947. The result was that growing support for assisted dying in The Netherlands, the U.S. and around the world stalled as countries attempted to distance themselves from Nazi Germany. The Nazi "euthanasia" programs set a pall over efforts to support voluntary euthanasia that continues to this day (Dowbiggin 2005:91–9; Kershaw 2001; Lifton 1986:51–79).

By the 1950s and '60s, a number of cases emerged that put assisted dying back on the radar in The Netherlands. In 1952, a doctor from Eindhoven was found guilty of killing his brother on request. His brother was dying of tuberculosis and had asked for help in dying. Although he could have received a jail sentence, the doctor was granted one year probation and the case came and went in the public domain with little notice (Griffiths, et al. 1998:44). In 1967, the Dutch public was presented with their first case of long term coma and euthanasia. Twenty-one year old Mia Versluis had been in a coma with severe and irreversible brain damage after cardiac arrest during a foot operation. A year later, Versluis' anesthe-siologist wanted to remove her feeding tube with the intention of ending her life. Her father fought this in court and the doctor was found guilty of "behavior that undermines confidence in the medical profession" (Griffiths, et al. 1998:48). He was fined 1000 guilders (roughly equivalent at that time to US $1500) and the court suggested that termination of life support should only be done if colleagues and family have been consulted.

A Physician-Led Movement. In 1969, Dutch psychiatrist and neurologist J. H. van den Berg confronted questions around the Versluis case and raised the concern for all physicians who had increasing medical ability to sustain life, but had not yet had the opportunity to discuss publicly whether life should be sustained. He argued that medical ethics must change with the times and what was a duty to preserve life at all costs, now must be a duty to preserve life whenever doing so makes sense. Van den Berg's book struck a nerve in The Netherlands, sparking a physician-led debate about the moral ethics of sustaining life. Meanwhile the cultural and legal climate in Holland was changing as well. By the 1970s, the Dutch reacted to a growing public liberalism against antiquated morality laws by legalizing abortion (1971) the sale of contraceptives (1970), and by repealing the crime of adultery (1971) and a restrictive provision on homosexuality (1971) (Griffiths, et al. 1998:45–49).

In the 1970s and early 1980s, public debates by physicians frustrated by the inadequacy of existing policies around end-of-life became more prominent. Dutch physicians began admitting publicly that they were providing their patients with assistance in dying, exposing a long understood bedside practice to the scrutiny of public debate. In addition, unlike in the U.S., the Royal Dutch Society for the Promotion of Health, formerly the Royal Dutch Medical Association (KNMG), came out in support of euthanasia and was instrumental in formulating the policy that resulted (Weyers 2006:806). In the beginning of these debates, "euthanasia" was used broadly to define a wide range of behaviors that shortened life. Physician debates and a handful of court cases during these decades, however, helped refine definitions, distinguishing Dutch "euthanasia" from other medical behaviors that potentially shorten life (MBPSL).[6]

In 1973, a physician terminated the life of her mother at her mother's request by giving her an injection of morphine. In the *Postma* case, the court found that giving increased doses of medication for pain relief, even if it is likely to cause death, does not constitute homicide. In 1981, the *Wertheim* case further delineated acceptable boundaries for euthanasia practice. In this case, a 67-year old woman was helped to die by a voluntary euthanasia activist. The activist was found guilty of assisted suicide and given a sentence of six months subject to one year probation due to Ms. Wertheim's age and limited physical condition. The court held that the decision to assist in a suicide must be done by a doctor and the doctor must not make the decision alone (Griffiths, et al. 1998:50–61).

Controlling Euthanasia. By 1982, the introduction of the *Schoonheim* case marked a turning point towards legalization of euthanasia. Dr. Schoonheim performed euthanasia on a 95-year old woman in the presence of her son, daughter-in-law and the doctor's assistant. The woman had a broken hip and was physically unable to walk, but mentally intact and had repeatedly asked her doctor for help in dying. Dr. Schoonheim was acquitted by the Dutch Supreme Court in 1984 on the basis that his actions followed from a "situation of necessity" where he had to choose between conflicting duties—his duty to relieve suffering versus a duty to respect life (Griffiths, et al. 1998:62–63). That same year, the KNMG issued a report outlining the Requirements for Due Care in cases

---

6. By the 1980s, euthanasia came to be defined as voluntary (at the patient's explicit request) and direct (an explicit act by the physician with intent to end life). Passive euthanasia has become known as "medical behavior that contributes to the end of life" and includes both withdrawing and withholding care as well as unintentional (indirect) death as a result of increased pain relief (e.g., death due to increased doses of morphine). See (Griffiths, et al. 1998:60).

of euthanasia or assisted suicide, helping to pave the way for legalized practice by Dutch physicians (Griffiths, et al. 1998:67–70). Since 1984, physicians could perform euthanasia or assisted suicide under the Requirements for Due Care in The Netherlands and not be prosecuted. The 1980s and 1990s saw several failed attempts at a euthanasia bill before the successful passing of the *Termination of Life on Request and Assisted Suicide (Review Procedures) Act* under a liberal majority government in 2001. With the passing of the Act, the Dutch formally de-criminalized euthanasia and assisted suicide by making the following changes to their Criminal Code. Prior to the 2001 changes, Articles 293 and 294 read,

Any person who terminates another person's life at that person's express and earnest request shall be liable to a term of imprisonment not exceeding twelve years or a fifth-category fine (Article 293).

Any person who intentionally incites another to commit suicide shall, if suicide follows, be liable to a term of imprisonment not exceeding three years or a fourth-category fine (Article 294).

After April 1, 2002, Articles 293 and 294 of the Dutch Criminal Code were revised to read,

1. Any person who terminates another person's life at that person's express and earnest request shall be liable to a term of imprisonment not exceeding twelve years or a fifth-category fine.

2. The act referred to in the first paragraph shall not be an offence if it committed by a physician who fulfils the due care criteria set out in Article 2 of the Termination of Life on Request and Assisted Suicide (Review Procedures) Act, and if the physician notifies the municipal pathologist of this act in accordance with the provisions of Article 7, paragraph 2 of the Burial and Cremation Act. (Article 293, The Act 2002); and

3. Any person who intentionally incites another to commit suicide shall, if suicide follows, be liable to a term of imprisonment not exceeding three years or a fine of the fourth-category fine.

4. Any person who intentionally assists another to commit suicide or provides him with the means to do so shall, if suicide follows, be liable to a term of imprisonment not exceeding three years or a fourth-category fine. Article 293, paragraph 2 shall apply mutatis mutandis (Article 294, The Act 2002).

Under the new law, physicians who perform euthanasia or assisted suicide are required to follow the statutory Requirements for Due Care and to report their actions to the coroner who will forward the information on to a regional review (*toetsing*) committee for an after-the-fact review. The Requirements of Due Care state that persons as young as 12 years old may request euthanasia or assisted suicide.[7] Persons 16 or older may receive euthanasia even if they are "no longer capable of expressing [their] will" if there is a prior written statement containing a request for termination of life.[8] Under Article 2 of the Act, euthanasia and assisted suicide must always be performed by a physician who:

a. holds the conviction that the request by the patient was voluntary and well-considered,

b. holds the conviction that the patient's suffering was lasting and unbearable,

---

7. According to Article 2 of Chapter II, Requirements for Due Care of the Act, "if the minor patient is aged between twelve and sixteen years and may be deemed to have a reasonable understanding of his interests, the physician may carry out the patient's request, provided always that the parent or the parents exercising parental authority and/or his guardian agree with the termination of life or the assisted suicide" (The Act 2002).

8. There are at least three different types of advanced directives in use in The Netherlands: (1) the euthanasia declaration, (2) the refusal of treatment document and (3) the do not resuscitate document (NVVE 2004).

c. has informed the patient about the situation he was in and about his prospects,

d. and the patient hold the conviction that there was no other reasonable solution for the situation he was in,

e. has consulted at least one other, independent physician who has seen the patient and has given his written opinion on the requirements of due care, referred to in parts a–d, and

f. has terminated a life or assisted in a suicide with due care (Requirements for Due Care, Article 2, The Act 2002).

For a complete copy of the *Termination of Life on Request and Assisted Suicide (Review Procedures) Act* (2002), see Appendix B.

Effective April 1, 2002, the Act changed little in terms of daily practice. Physicians in The Netherlands still follow virtually the same requirements of due care outlined prior to the 2002 Act and government debates still center around palliative care, euthanasia reporting frequencies, and cases that define the borders of legal practice. The shift was largely symbolic, the end of a period of legal development, but making little in the way of changes to current practice.

Other Medical Behaviors that Potentially Shorten Life. Periodically international concerns of the presence of a "slippery slope" at work in The Netherlands emerge, often prompted by reports of euthanasia cases for reasons other than terminal illness, liberal attitudes towards infant euthanasia, or speculation on making a suicide pill (the Drion Pill) widely available to Dutch citizens (Chabot 2007; Sheldon 2004; Verhagen and Sauer 2005). One of the more enduring criticisms of Dutch euthanasia, the "slippery slope" argument, is premised on the belief that allowing physicians to assist in legal suicide or euthanasia for persons who are incurably ill may lead to situations in which healthy patients are killed against their will (Battin 2005). With the experience of Nazi Germany still so close at hand, this argument remains one of the more powerful criticisms of the Dutch experience with euthanasia and other medical behavior that potentially shorten life (MBPSL).

To respond to worldwide criticism by opponents of the policy, the Dutch government formed the Remmelink Commission to study euthanasia and other related medical behaviors at the end of life. In 1990, the van der Wal and van der Maas study (originally called the Remmelink study) estimated that the number of euthanasia and assisted suicide cases in The Netherlands was 1.7 and 0.2 percent of all deaths, respectively, a relatively low figure in relation to all deaths. But we know from this time that not all physicians were regularly reporting euthanasia cases and in addition to this figure, there were a number of deaths that raised some concern. Approximately 18.8 percent of all deaths were cases in which death occurred following an increase of medication to alleviate pain symptoms, 17.9 percent of all deaths that year were cases in which life-prolonging treatments were withheld or withdrawn (WH/WD) and approximately 0.8 percent of deaths fell under a category of life-terminating acts without the explicit request of the patient (LAWER). The majority of LAWER cases included patients who were close to death, no longer able to communicate, and appeared to be suffering severely (Griffiths, et al. 2008:181).

Since this first study, there have been three follow-up studies. These studies revealed an increase in euthanasia and WH/WD in 1995 and 2001 and then a drop in both categories in 2005. LAWER cases held steady until 2001, after which these dropped from 0.7 percent to 0.4 percent. Pain relief with life-shortening effect has increased steadily since 1990, with the largest gain in 2005. In 2005, the study also identified 8.2 percent of all deaths in which continuous, deep sedation prior to death had occurred (van der Heide, et al. 2007). See Table 3.1.

Initially, LAWER cases and other MBPSL cases with intention by the physician to shorten life were seen by many outsiders as cause for concern, sparking a number of responses suggesting that these and other cases are examples of a "slippery slope" in existence in The Netherlands (Gillick MD 2004; Hendin 1997; Keown 1995; Kuhse 1992). American physician Muriel Gillick suggested recently that some forms of MBPSL may very well be euthanasia in disguise. Using secondary data from an interview study of 410 Dutch physicians (Rietjens, et al. 2004), Gillick argues that the practice of ter-

Table 3.1 Euthanasia and Other Medical Behavior That Potentially Shortens Life (MBPSL) as a Percentage of All Deaths in The Netherlands, 1990–2005

	1990	1995	2001	2005
Euthanasia*	1.7	2.4	2.6	1.7
Assisted suicide*	0.2	0.2	0.2	0.1
Discussed with patient (or previous patient wish)			100.0	100.0
Discussed with relative of patient			96.0	75.5
Shortening of life by <1 week			45.9	44.8
Life-terminating acts without explicit request by the patient (LAWER)*	0.8	0.7	0.7	0.4
Discussed with patient (or previous patient wish)			26.5	60.0
Discussed with relative of patient			100.0	80.9
Discussed with ≥1 other physician			65.2	65.3
Shortening of life by <1 week			77.3	85.5
Pain relief with life-shortening effect*	18.8	19.1	20.1	24.7
Subsidiary intention to hasten death**	4	3	2	1
Withholding or withdrawing of life-prolonging treatment (WH/WD)*	17.9	20.2	20.2	15.6
Express intention to hasten death**	9	13	13	8
Continuous deep sedation*	NA	NA	NA	8.2
Terminal sedation **				>1.0
Auto-euthanasia***	NA	NA	3.2	NA
Suicide by stopping with eating/drinking			2.1	
Suicide by overdose			1.1	

* See van der Heide et al. 2007. End-of-life practices in The Netherlands under the Euthanasia Act. *The New England Journal of Medicine* 356(19):1957, Tables 1 and 3.

** See Griffiths, Weyers, and Adams 2008. Euthanasia and Law in Europe. Oxford, UK: Hart Publishing, pp. 154, 177.

*** See Chabot, Boudewijn 2007. Auto-Euthanasie: Verborgen Stervenswegen in Gesprek met Naasten. Amsterdam: Bert Bakker, p. 106.

minal sedation (the administration of sedating medications with cessation of nutrition and hydration) reveals some disturbing trends. Gillick was concerned by physicians' intention to hasten death, by the low number of explicit requests for terminal sedation by the patients, and by a lack of palliative care alternatives. According to the Rietjens study on which Gillick's argument is based, nearly two-thirds of Dutch physicians stated that they intended to hasten death or both hasten death and alleviate symptoms, 59 percent of patients discussed terminal sedation with their physician, 33 percent specifically requested deep sedation, and specialists in palliative care were "rarely" consulted (Rietjens, et al. 2004).

American physician Herbert Hendin and his colleagues (Foley and Hendin 2002) also take aim at some of the figures on Dutch end-of-life, suggesting that the 1990 and 1995 studies revealed approximately 4,813 (3.7 percent) and 6,368 (4.7 percent) total deaths that can be viewed as 'nonvoluntary,' which they define as "euthanasia with patients not capable of requesting it," or 'involuntary,' "euthanasia with patients who did not request it but were capable of doing so." Hendin includes in these figures cases of euthanasia, assisted suicide, LAWER cases, and an additional number of cases where opioids were given by a physician with the explicit intention of ending life (Hendin 2002:97–106). Griffiths and his colleagues (2008) disagree. They argue that while many of the "acts and omissions that a doctor engages in during the course of treating a patient violate the literal terms of provisions of the criminal law prohibiting causing bodily harm," the Dutch Penal code has since its inception included an implicit medical exception for physicians (Griffiths, et al. 2008:54). Medical exceptions are considered "normal medical practice" and fall under the scope of professional standards set by the KNMG. These include the refusal of treatments and advanced directives, withholding or withdrawal of life-prolonging treatments based on medical futility, the administration of pain relief that may contribute to death, palliative and terminal sedation. Euthanasia and assisted suicide are not considered to be "normal medical practice," but are covered by the *Termination of Life on Request (Review Procedures) Act* (2002).

As Griffiths and colleagues point out, much of the debate around MBPSL has been driven by a focus on the intention of the physician to hasten death. According to Griffiths et al., however, "as far as the law in concerned, it is the fact that pain relief is *medically indicated,* and not the doctor's subjective intention, that protects the doctor from criminal liability" (Griffiths, et al. 2008:64). Because intention has been such a focus of data collection, Griffiths et al. can calculate that the percentage of deaths *intentionally* caused by physicians in 2005 was 11 percent, compared to 16 percent in 1990, 19 percent in 1995 and 17 percent in 2001. This includes all euthanasia, PAS, and LAWER cases, as well as pain relief with a subsidiary intention to hasten death, and WH/WD with an express intention to hasten death (Griffiths, et al. 2008:153).

Proponents of euthanasia policy argue that these cases need to be examined more closely, that essentially not all LAWER and MBPSL cases are created equal. According to Griffiths et al. (2008), many MBPSL rates are similar to rates found in other European countries, including rates of abstention, withdrawing or withholding treatments, pain relief with life shortening effects, and termination of life without the patient's explicit request (Griffiths, et al. 2008:158). Pijnenborg and van der Maas (1993) suggest that in a country where 99.4 percent of the population has comprehensive healthcare insurance and 100 percent are covered for the costs of long-term illness, end-of-life patients are not vulnerable due to lack of financial resources for care. In addition, their original 1990 study revealed that in 59 percent of all LAWER cases, patients had made their end-of-life wishes known to the physician (just short of an explicit request). In 70 percent of these cases the physician had consulted a colleague and in 83 percent they had consulted with relatives. Physicians knew their patients on the average of 2.4 years (for specialists) and 7.2 years (for general practitioners) and in 86 percent of all LAWER cases life was shortened only by a few hours or days (Pijnenborg and van der Maas 1993). By 2001, it was estimated that 26.5 of all LAWER cases were based on a previous communication with the patient, 100 percent included consultation with relatives, 65 percent included consultation with one or more other physicians, and in more than 77 percent of LAWER cases it was estimated that life was shortened by less than a week. By 2005, those figures remained fairly similar except that as many as 60 percent included a previous communication with the patient, almost 90 percent included consultation with relatives and in over 85 percent of LAWER cases in 2005 it was estimated that life was shortened by less than a week (van der Heide, et al. 2007:1957). See Table 3.1.

In The Netherlands, there is a relatively new category of MBPSL that is raising concern. This is terminal sedation, sometimes also called palliative or continuous deep sedation (Battin 2008; Gillick 2004; Griffiths, et al. 2008:66–71, 176–177; Tännsjö 2004). Battin (2008) suggests that recent attempts by the American Medical Association to differentiate between terminal sedation and euthanasia in the U.S. are problematic. She argues that while there are morally defensible pros and cons to terminal sedation, without clear guidelines and safeguards even humane practices that may fall under this category of MBPSL become morally problematic. Griffiths and colleagues (2008) suggest that the term needs to be better defined. They define terminal sedation as a potential cause of death due to sedation accompanied by withholding of artificial nutrition or hydration for a period long enough that it can be expected to hasten death. They suggest it is important to distinguish terminal sedation from palliative sedation, which they define as "putting a patient into deep sleep, in the expectation that this will be continued until his death" (Griffiths, et al. 2008:66). Terminal and palliative sedation have drawn increasing attention in The Netherlands with their inclusion in the 2005 van der Wal and van der Maas study. In 2005, the KNMG came out with guidelines on palliative sedation, deeming deep, continuous sedation until death and the withholding of artificial nutrition and hydration as "normal medical practices." While these guidelines offer a good first step in regulating behavior that falls under this umbrella term, Griffiths et al. argue that in order to ensure that terminal sedation does not become an unregulated alternative to euthanasia, further regulation specifically on terminal sedation as they define it is needed.

Griffiths et al. suggest that terminal sedation accounted for less than 1 percent of all deaths in 2005 (Griffiths, et al. 2008:66–71, 177).

A final category of behavior at the end of life that is raising concern is a practice termed, "auto-euthanasia." Dutch researcher and psychologist Boudewijn Chabot (2007) published a study of auto-euthanasia, a term he uses to describe a type of suicide that occurs by patients mostly for medical reasons done in consultation with one or more persons, but without physician assistance or authorization. In each of the cases he examined, an end-of-life association was consulted. Chabot examined two types of deaths: auto-euthanasia by cessation of eating and drinking and auto-euthanasia by lethal drug overdose. In his study, Chabot estimates that between 1999 and 2003, an average of 3.2 percent of all deaths each year can be attributed to either auto-euthanasia by stopping eating and drinking (2.1 percent) or by a lethal dose of sleeping pills (1.1 percent) (Chabot 2007:106). Chabot examined 144 cases of auto-euthanasia for specific characteristics. He found that almost half of all cases occurred after denial of a request for euthanasia by a physician (49 percent), a number of cases that indicated psychiatric illness (10 percent)[9] or no serious illness at all (26 percent), and a large number of cases where it was predicted the patient would have lived one month or more (79 percent) (Chabot 2007:121, 131, 133). Compared to my sample, Chabot's cases largely appear to be the kind of cases that *huisartsen* tend to avoid. According to Griffiths et al., it is estimated that approximately 10 percent of all deaths in The Netherlands each year include a person's exercising "some degree of control over the timing and manner of death, without this taking the socially-isolated and often violent form of suicide" (Griffiths, et al. 2008:182). This includes estimates on euthanasia, PAS, auto-euthanasia, terminal sedation and WH/WD treatment at the request of the patient.

---

9. The percentage of psychiatric illness cases can be calculated by adding the number of psychiatric diagnoses with stopping with eating and drinking cases (n=5) with overdose by sleeping pills (n=10) divided by the total number of auto-euthanasia cases (n=144).

Dutch Health Care System. The Dutch policy on euthanasia and assisted suicide is situated in a system of healthcare that is quite different from that in the U.S. Persons who are nearing the end of life or who live with chronic illness have an extensive array of services that are available. During my study, the Dutch insurance system consisted of public and private sector funding streams that gave coverage to almost 100 percent of the population. Anyone below a certain salary (€31,750 gross per year in 2003) was covered by *Ziekenfonds*, the government subsidized, but privately managed, insurance system that covered approximately two-thirds of the population. The Dutch system makes a distinction between normal medical costs and long-term, high-costs, covering these "exceptional" costs through government funding. The *Algemene Wet Bijzondere Ziektekosten* (AWBZ) or General Law for Extraordinary Medical Costs is available to everyone to cover the cost of nursing home care, some home care, and medical equipment. In 2006 in The Netherlands, approximately 72.2 percent of the cost of health care was covered by social health insurance, 8 percent was paid for by patients, 6.8 percent by private insurance, and an additional 13 percent by government and other unspecified sources. Social health insurance also covered approximately 66.8 percent of welfare costs (including extraordinary medical costs for persons who are elderly or disabled), 11.8 were paid for by patients, and 21.4 were covered by government and other unspecified sources (CBS 2007:99–100). On January 1, 2006, the Dutch passed healthcare reform, changing to a single, compulsory system of national health care insurance for all. It is a new system of "managed competition," which keeps general practitioners as the gatekeepers, but allows consumers freedom now to change their insurer and insurance plan. (Griffiths, et al. 2008:15–23; Grol 2006; Weel 2004).

Thuiszorg is the national Dutch homecare association which provides assistance in the home up to four times per day including assistance with personal care, meals, medications, nursing care, and overnight respite (in which a nursing assistant spends the night to care for the patient as needed and to give the family time to sleep). In addition, there are services that deliver home-cooked meals and come by regularly to clean the house. I worked with *Amsterdam Thuiszorg* and the level of home care services available to persons in The Netherlands with chronic or life-threatening illness is really quite amazing, even despite the waiting lists that some experience. Persons who are terminally ill are typically moved up on waitlists and everyone in my study who needed home-based services was able to receive them. Even those patients who were no longer able to get out of bed, were fully incontinent, or required daily nursing care were able to stay at home with the assistance of *Thuiszorg*.

If someone requires more than either *Thuiszorg* or family members can provide in the home, then the choice must be made to move to one of several types of long-term or acute care facilities for which there are also waitlists. Many end-of-life patients I met spent time in and out of the hospital (*ziekenhuis*). For those with minimal needs, there are independent living apartments (*aanleunwoning*) where residents have access to nursing and personal care services but have their own apartment with a kitchen where they can live alone or with a partner. There are residential or nursing homes (*verzorgingshuizen*) and elder care homes (*bejaardenhuizen*), where residents have rooms, typically without kitchens that are situated off a hallway staffed by nurses and nurse assistants. Like the *aanleunwoning*, residents tend to decorate their own apartment using furniture from home, but in these units they have more access to nursing and personal care. Persons living in any of these locations also keep their own *huisarts* and many of the house calls I went on were to persons living in these types of homes.

If 24-hour care is needed, there is the acute care nursing facility (*verpleeghuis*) or in a few places, like Amsterdam, hospice is available to those who are at the end of life. *Verpleeghuizen* will have any number of units, some devoted to persons living with dementia and some for palliative care at the end of life. Compared to the U.S. and most notably Britain, hospice is not prominent in The Netherlands. Instead, it appears that where hospice was added to supplement palliative care services in end of life care in the U.S. and elsewhere, these same services were largely not missed in the current Dutch health care system, where families are given quite a bit of support to die at home and *huisartsen* are much more in-volved than many of their U.S. counterparts in providing pallia-tive care at the end of life. In 2003, approximately one third of all persons who died in The Netherlands that year died in the hospi-tal; more than one-quarter died at home and one-fifth died in ei-ther a residential/nursing, elder care or acute care nursing facility (*verzorgingshuis, bejaardenhuis,* or *verpleeghuis*) (CBS 2004).

The American Experience

Where in The Netherlands assisted dying has largely been a physi-cian-led movement with the focus on euthanasia practice, in the U.S., it is a patient-rights movement that continues to be domi-nated by religious conservatives typically taking the pro-life stance and an often splintered group of patient's rights advocates taking the right-to-die stance. In the U.S., the tension between patients and the medical system has evolved into a much more contentious doctor-patient relationship that does not typically include house calls nor increased involvement by the physician once efforts at treatment are shifted towards palliative care. While there are states and local regions that are better equipped to assist families at the end of life, there is no cohesive system of end-of-life care at this time in the U.S. The following details key events in recent history that mark the current state of assisted dying in the United States.

A Patient's Rights Movement. Public interest in euthanasia first peaked in the late 1930s with the founding of the Euthanasia Soci-ety of America by wealthy New Yorker, Ann Mitchell, and ex-Uni-tarian minister, Charles Potter aided by several high profile cases of "mercy killing" in the press. Just as in most of Europe, interest in euthanasia waned in the aftermath of Hitler's *Aktion T4* program and the Holocaust. In the 1970s and '80s, interest in assisted dying peaked again as a part of a patient's rights movement. This move-ment followed the turbulent aftermath of the Vietnam War and a growing collective consciousness that set individual rights in op-position to state and medical authority. That coupled with the increased ability of medical science to prolong life and the relative disappearance of religion at the bedside of the dying, led families to question whether life *should be* prolonged and who—patients, doctors or families—had the right to decide.

In 1972, trustees of the American Hospital Association drew up the first Patient's Bill of Rights, which outlined patient's rights to informed consent and the right of patients to refuse treatment (Starr 1982:390). In 1974, the Society for the Right to Die (formerly the Euthanasia Society of America) re-formed and the first hospice in the U.S. opened in Connecticut. In 1976, the case of 21 year old Karen Ann Quinlan raised public concern for patients caught in a persistent vegetative state and the doctor's requirement to continue treatment. After a night of drinking and drug use, Karen Quinlan collapsed into a coma at a roadside bar and for almost a year after, her family fought for the right to withdraw her from life-sustaining treatment. The family eventually won their case and Quinlan died nine years after being disconnected from the respirator (Dowbiggin 2005:121–22).

In 1980, the Hemlock Society was formed by Derek Humphry, a Los Angeles-based British journalist who helped his wife die and then wrote a book about it (Humphry 1978). In 1981 the first case of AIDS was identified in the U.S., which eventually led to an underground assisted dying movement among gay communities across the nation. In 1989, the Nancy Cruzan case was heard by the U.S. Supreme Court, which ruled that the Constitution supports a patient's right to refuse treatment if there is "clear and convincing evidence" of the refusal. Nancy Cruzan was 25 years old and suffered severe cognitive and physical disabilities following a car crash. She was completely incapacitated by her accident but was not in a coma or on a respirator. Her parents fought for the right to withdraw treatment and in 1990 Cruzan died 12 days after artificial administration of food and fluids were withdrawn (Dowbiggin 2005:134–35). Today, the threat of lawsuits against doctors and the cost of medical malpractice insurance shapes American medicine in ways that does not occur elsewhere. The doctor-patient-family relationship remains a contentious one.

A Conflicted Movement. American debates around assisted dying have been marked by conflict, both polarization between right-to-die and pro-life advocates and lack of cohesion by those advocating for assisted dying policy. By the 1990s, assistance in dying became a legislative concern in the U.S. There were a number of events that marked this period of time. Right-to-die organizations formed and re-formed, marked by some successes and a lot of infighting. By its height in the mid-1990s, the Hemlock Society, probably the best known right-to-die organization in the U.S., had as many as 46,000 members and was active in raising awareness of right-to-die issues as well as drafting and promoting right-to-die legislation across the country. As momentum grew so did the conflicts. Factions split off and merged again and with so many mergers and name changes, cohesion during this time was lost. End-of-Life Choices was based in Colorado and Compassion in Dying based in Washington State. In 2003, the Hemlock Society merged with the Colorado-based group, but a year later original Hemlock members unhappy with the merger formed their own organization, the Final Exit Network. In 2005, Compassion in Dying and End-of-Life Choices merged, becoming Compassion & Choices (Compassion & Choices 2005; Humphry 2005; Scherer and Simon 1999:33–5).

In the 1990s, Jack Kevorkian (pathologist turned right-to-die advocate, also known in the media as "Dr. Death") gained notoriety for assisting in the deaths of as many as 130 persons, some of whom were disabled and not terminally ill. In 1994 and again in 1996, Kevorkian was acquitted of assisting several suicides. In 1998, Kevorkian stunned viewers of CBS' *60 Minutes* when he performed the second televised euthanasia death on national television.[10] View-

---

10. This case was different than earlier reported cases of assisted suicide by Kevorkian because in this case, Kevorkian injected the man with lethal drugs as opposed to providing the person with the means to kill themselves. The legal difference is that, unlike assisted suicide, euthanasia in the U.S. is tried as a murder case where evidence of suffering and com-

ers watched as Kevorkian killed a 52 year old man suffering from end-stage Lou Gehrig's disease. In 1999, Kevorkian was convicted of second degree murder for this and served eight years of a 10 to 25 year sentence (AP 2007; Garsten 1999; Scherer and Simon 1999:28–9). As a spokesman for the right-to-die movement, Kevorkian did his followers no favors by advocating such an extremist stance that he often alienated mainstream supporters of assistance in dying.

In 1991, Derek Humphry published *Final Exit*, a how-to on suicide which shot to the best-seller list and soon became a manual for those around the world who sought a humane and certain method outside of the law for assisted dying (Humphry 1991). Unfortunately however, Humphry's suggested method of drug overdose combined with asphyxiation (a plastic bag over the head) while effective is probably not the most peaceful way to die, nor an easy passing for the family or loved ones to witness. Regardless, by the 1990s, *Final Exit* was brought into use as the AIDS epidemic began claiming more and more lives. Dying from complications due to AIDS can be a horrible way to die with protracted suffering and multiple painful and debilitating conditions. Isolated from mainstream society, networks of gay men began to make their own rules for death and dying. The rates of suicide among gay men in the 1980s and early '90s skyrocketed; it was not unusual for men dying of AIDS to bequeath their stash of lethal pills to someone else who was dying and a number of organizations, like Safe Passages in Los Angeles, emerged to provide assistance in dying for men stricken with HIV/AIDS (Dowbiggin 2005:134; Shavelson 1995:35–67).

From 1998 to 2005, the Terri Schiavo case made headlines. Schiavo was just 26 years old when she suffered irreversible brain damage due to complications from an "iced tea diet" and years of damage

---

passion is not deemed relevant. The first televised euthanasia death was performed by Dutch general practitioner, Dr. van Oijen, in 1994.

from bulimia. She lay in a persistent vegetative state (awake, eyes open, but without awareness) for a year before her husband petitioned for the right to remove her feeding tube. What ensued was an almost seven year battle between her husband, her parents (who opposed withdrawing life support), and the Florida legal system. Fueled by the media, the Schiavo case tapped into deep-seated concepts of who has the right to decide (married partners versus blood relatives) and life (consciousness versus brain death), sparking the interest of the Florida governor, Jeb Bush (and brother to the President); U.S. Congress; and eventually President George W. Bush. After several attempts at state and federal legislation to block Schiavo's husband from withdrawing support, the Florida court determined that Terri Schiavo's wishes prior to her illness were to not continue life-prolonging measures and in March 2005, her feeding tube was removed. She died 13 days later after which the autopsy revealed that her brain was approximately half the size of a healthy human brain (NNDB 2008).

In 2005, a physician and two nurses made headlines after allegedly performing euthanasia on a number of hospital patients when they found themselves without electricity, clean water or imminent rescue in the aftermath of Hurricane Katrina in New Orleans (Griffin and Johnston 2006). Even though the patients appeared to be near the end of life and suffering due to inadequate conditions caused by the storm, the public outcry was mostly against hospital staff who would allow euthanasia to happen even under these extreme conditions. In 2007, two nurses charged were offered immunity in exchange for their testimony. The physician in the case was charged with 10 counts, including second-degree murder and conspiracy to commit second-degree murder. In July 2007, a Louisiana grand jury decided not to indict the physician on criminal charges, although several civil suits are still pending (Jalsevac 2007).

Legalization at the State-Level. The fight to legalize assisted dying in the U.S. has largely occurred at the state level. Since the 19th century, as many as 44 U.S. states have had statutes or laws on the books prohibiting assisted suicide. By the late 1990s and early 2000s, laws for and against assisted dying came to the forefront in the U.S. In 1994, state bans on physician-assisted suicide were challenged in Washington and New York states. In 1997, the Supreme Court ruled that there is no constitutional right for physician-assisted suicide, leaving it up to the states to decide their own laws (Scherer and Simon 1999:39–40). Between 1990 and 2008, a number of states attempted to pass legislation for assisted dying by ballot measures in California (1992), Maine (2000), Michigan (1998) and Washington state (1991 and 2008) and by legislative bills in 21 states, including most notably Arizona, California, Hawaii, Michigan, Oregon, Vermont and Wisconsin (Dunsmuir and Tiedemann 2007; ITF 2007).

Today, physician-assisted dying is legal in two states: Oregon (since 1997) and most recently Washington (since 2008). In Oregon, the *Death With Dignity Act* (1997), on which many of these later bills are modeled, was passed and upheld despite regular attempts by religious conservatives to overturn the law. The law passed by voter ballot with a slim margin in 1994, but due to appeals did not go into effect until November 1997. In June 1997, the Oregon legislature in response to challenges regarding the Act, sent it back to the voters to decide and they again voted to keep it, this time by a vote of 60 to 40 percent.

Since 1997, "an adult who is capable, is a resident of Oregon, and has been determined by the attending physician and consulting physician to be suffering from a terminal disease, and who has voluntarily expressed his or her wish to die, may make a written request [to a physician] for medication for the purpose of ending his or her life" (ORS 127.800 to 127.897 1997). The attending physician must:

> (a) Make the initial determination of whether a patient has a terminal disease, is capable, and has made the request voluntarily;
> (b) Request that the patient demonstrate Oregon residency pursuant to ORS 127.860;
> (c) To ensure that the patient is making an informed decision, inform the patient of:

(A) His or her medical diagnosis;

(B) His or her prognosis;

(C) The potential risks associated with taking the medication to be prescribed;

(D) The probable result of taking the medication to be prescribed; and

(E) The feasible alternatives, including, but not limited to, comfort care, hospice care and pain control;

(d) Refer the patient to a consulting physician for medical confirmation of the diagnosis, and for a determination that the patient is capable and acting voluntarily;

(e) Refer the patient for counseling if appropriate pursuant to ORS 127.825;

(f) Recommend that the patient notify next of kin;

(g) Counsel the patient about the importance of having another person present when the patient takes the medication prescribed pursuant to ORS 127.800 to 127.897 and of not taking the medication in a public place;

(h) Inform the patient that he or she has an opportunity to rescind the request at any time and in any manner, and offer the patient an opportunity to rescind at the end of the 15 day waiting period pursuant to ORS 127.840;

(i) Verify, immediately prior to writing the prescription for medication under ORS 127.800 to 127.897, that the patient is making an informed decision;

(j) Fulfill the medical record documentation requirements of ORS 127.855;

(k) Ensure that all appropriate steps are carried out in accordance with ORS 127.800 to 127.897 prior to writing a prescription for medication to enable a qualified patient to end his or her life in a humane and dignified manner; and

(l) (A) Dispense medications directly, including ancillary medications intended to facilitate the desired

effect to minimize the patient's discomfort, provided
the attending physician is registered as a dispensing
physician with the Board of Medical Examiners, has
a current Drug Enforcement Administration certificate and complies with any applicable administrative rule; or

(B) With the patient's written consent:

(i) Contact a pharmacist and inform the pharmacist of the prescription; and

(ii) Deliver the written prescription personally or
by mail to the pharmacist, who will dispense the
medications to either the patient, the attending
physician or an expressly identified agent of the
patient. [1995 c.3 §3.01; 1999 c.423 §3][11]

The Catholic Church, pro-life organizations, such as the National
Right to Life Committee founded in 1973, and disability advocates, such as Not Dead Yet, have been the most vocal against assisted dying policy in the U.S. (NDY n.d.; NRLC n.d.; PFL n.d.).
In 2001, Senator John Ashcroft attempted to have the controlled
substance licenses of physicians who prescribe lethal doses of controlled substances under the Oregon law revoked, stating that
physicians were violating the *Controlled Substance Act* of 1970.
Then Attorney General Janet Reno declared that the *Controlled
Substance Act* does not authorize the Drug Enforcement Administration (DEA) to revoke the registration of a physician who has
"assisted in a suicide in compliance with the Oregon law." In 2001,
newly appointed attorney general Ashcroft issued a directive attempting to suspend or revoke DEA registration of Oregon physicians who perform assisted suicide. The matter went to court and
in 2006 the Supreme Court affirmed the lower courts' decisions
to uphold the Oregon *Death with Dignity Act,* ruling that former

---

11. For a complete copy of the *Oregon Death with Dignity Act,* see Appendix C.

Table 3.2 Percentage and Number of Physician-Assisted Deaths (PAD) in Oregon, 1998–2007

	1998	2001	2005	2007
Termination of life on request PAD	16	21	32	49
Requests for PAD Legal prescriptions requested	24	44	64	85
Ratio of PAD to 10,000 total deaths Legal prescription requests*	5.5% 66.7%	7.1% 47.7%	12.0% 50.0%	15.6% 57.6%
Total deaths	Unknown	Unknown	Unknown	Unknown

* Computed by dividing number of PAD by number of legal prescriptions.

Source: (DHS 2008; Leman, et al. 2006:4–5) This is a partial list of figures available for each year from 1998 to 2007.

attorney general Ashcroft acted without legal authority in his 2001 directive (Greenhouse 2006; NCSL 2008).

To date, not many citizens of Oregon have chosen to die by physician-assisted dying (PAD). The figure each year is so small that researchers typically measure the ratio of PAD per 10,000 deaths. In 2003, however, it was reported that less than 1/7 of one percent of Oregonians died by PAD (Leman and Hopkins 2004:5). Although we do not have the number of total deaths each year for Oregon, it is clear from the 2003 report that the ratio of PAD to total deaths is much lower in Oregon where the policy is also much younger—1997 in Oregon versus 1984 in The Netherlands (see Tables 2.1 and 3.2).

Looking at the number of euthanasia/PAS deaths to concrete requests (requests typically made after serious diagnosis of illness) in The Netherlands and the number of PAD to lethal prescriptions requested in Oregon, we can make some limited comparisons regarding termination of life requests initiated and concrete requests made. Looking at Figure 3.1, we find that persons who make serious requests for PAD in Oregon have a higher likelihood of dying with physician assistance than do their Dutch counterparts. In its first year, 66.7 percent of those who initiated requests for a lethal prescription with their physician in Oregon went through with an assisted death. That figure dropped somewhat in 2001 (47.7 percent) and 2005 (50 percent) and rose in 2007 (57.6 percent). Still we can say that between half to three-fifths of all requests for PAD in Oregon end in an assisted death. This suggests the possibility of some similarities between The Netherlands and Oregon regarding the difference between talking about assisted dying versus going through with it.

Between 1997 and 2007, a total of 341 persons have died by physician assisted suicide in the state of Oregon. As in previous years, most recent figures indicate that most were between the ages of 55 and 84 years of age (80 percent) with a median age of 65, most died at home (90 percent) and were enrolled in hospice (88 percent) and the majority had terminal cancer (86 percent). The reasons given for choosing PAD were loss of autonomy (100 percent), decreased ability to participate in activities that made life enjoyable (86 percent) and loss of dignity (86 percent) (DHS 2008).

Figure 3.1 Percentage of Persons who Initiated Concrete Requests and Died Euthanasia/PAS Deaths in The Netherlands versus Percentage of Persons who Initiated Prescription Requests and Died Physician-Assisted Deaths in Oregon, USA*

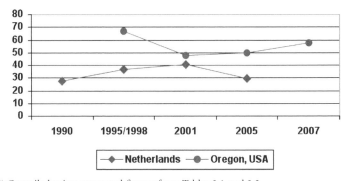

* Compiled using computed figures from Tables 2.1 and 3.2.

American Health Care System. Advanced directives, patient's rights and assisted dying arose within the context of a unique system of healthcare in the U.S. Compared to 30 industrialized nations from around the world, the U.S. is the *only* industrialized nation without universal health coverage (Vladeck 2003). The U.S. has the highest per capita cost of health care in the world, yet 46.6 million people (15.9 percent of the population) remain uninsured (OECD 2006; U.S. Census 2006; WHO 2007). Compared to the Dutch system, the coverage for end-of-life care is limited in the U.S., particularly if you cannot afford to pay for it yourself.

In 1935, the Social Security Act was passed after much debate and without the inclusion of national health coverage due in part to opposition by the American Medical Association (AMA). The Social Security Act provides financial assistance for the elderly and working poor, but today Social Security is under threat as policy analysts predict that without reform, the growing number of elderly recipients will increase beyond what the current fund can sustain as early as the year 2041 (GAO 2005:19; Starr 1982:266–275). In 1965, President Johnson signed Medicare and Medicaid into law, again measures opposed by the increasingly powerful AMA. Medicare and Medicaid were formed to cover hospital and physician costs for the elderly and the poor. In 1981, freedom of choice waivers and Home- and Community-Based waivers were added to the Medicaid program allowing Medicaid funds to be used for home supports for persons who are low-income and elderly or living with chronic disabilities. In 2003, a prescription drug benefit was added to Medicare under President George W. Bush (CMS n.d.). In 2005, the Deficit Reduction Act allowed funds for states to enact Money Follows the Person (MFP) grants to develop more comprehensive systems of community-based, long term care (CMS 2008). Medicaid is the main government program that pays for long term care in the U.S. and continues to be a program that favors institutional care, even for those who do not require it, over home- and community-based supports (Gleckman 2009:145–170).

Today, the cost burden of U.S. healthcare falls predominantly to private business and individual citizens. Only 44.7 percent of the total expenditure on healthcare is covered by the U.S. government, compared to, for example, 62.4 percent coverage in The Netherlands, 86.3 percent in the UK, and 69.8 percent in Canada, all countries that have universal health coverage (WHO 2007:64, 68, 72). Talk of national health coverage came up again in the early 1990s during President Clinton's term in office and most recently in the democratic debates for the 2008 Presidential elections. In 1993, President Clinton's wife, First Lady Hillary Clinton, spearheaded the health care reform effort, stating, "here in America people are dying because they couldn't get the care they needed when they were sick. It's time to provide quality affordable health care for every American" (CNN 2007). But this was not to be. This time the AMA and the American Hospital Association did not oppose the employer mandate plan, but they also did not come out in support of it. Ultimately, a complicated plan and factions among interest groups and among Democrats supporting the various plans ended the prospects of universal coverage during the Clinton administration (Starr 1995). In 2008, discussions of universal coverage were again revived with the election of Barack Obama as U.S. President in November 2008. Obama ran on a platform that offered to ensure health coverage for all by guaranteeing eligibility and affordability of health insurance; by strengthening employer coverage; curtailing the influence of insurance and pharmaceutical companies, such as ending the ability of insurance carriers to cancel coverage based on pre-existing conditions and allowing consumers to purchase drugs overseas; and by strengthening preventive care (Obama and Biden 2007).

The focus on universal coverage is important because the current health care system to a large extent impacts how Americans are able to die in this country and exposes some real limitations in terms of patient choice at the end of life (Gleckman 2009; Kaufman 2005; Gass 2004; Diamond 1992). Even with Social Security Insurance, Medicare, and Medicaid, there are costs at the end of life for which there is no safety net. Medicare generally covers the first 100 days of skilled nursing and rehabilitation services and for hospice once a patient qualifies. Medicaid is only available to Americans who drop below a certain income level, which means that for many elderly Americans they will need to pay for their own care at home or in the nursing home until they die or until such time that their personal savings are depleted. According to the American Association for Retired Persons (AARP), the bulk of long-term care in this country is provided by family and friends, and the bulk of long-term care is paid for by personal savings accounts. One study estimates that as much as one-third of families of patients hospitalized with serious illness lost most or all of their personal savings as a result of costs not paid for by other sources (AARP n.d.; Covinsky, et al. 1994). Volunteer and faith-based organizations fill in some of the gaps. Local organizations will offer some services to the elderly, the poor, and the chronically ill and disabled, and hospice provides limited services on a sliding scale fee (or free of charge) to those with a terminal prognosis and an estimated six months or less left to live.

Just as in The Netherlands, most Americans today continue to die in the hospital even though that is often not the kind of death they say they want. According to medical anthropologist Sharon Kaufman (2005), the American tendency is to attempt to stave off death with the most sophisticated (and expensive) treatments and technologies. Kaufman states that as many as one-quarter of all hospitalized patients are treated in an intensive care unit of a hospital before they die and when they enter the hospital system they enter a system that due to a complex set of circumstances, including the ever prevalent threat of legal action against healthcare practitioners in the U.S., pushes life-saving treatments even when none of the participants (hospital staff, patients or families) view that as the best choice. The result is a way of dying that alienates all involved and as Kaufman describes is anything but "dignified" (Kaufman 2005).

Palliative and hospice care is on the rise in the U.S. and is beginning to offer some real alternatives to death in the hospital. Palliative care units that focus on offering comfort and care to both patients and families at the very end of life are being added to hospitals across the country. In 1982, Medicare changed its benefits to include coverage for hospice, which provides home-based nursing, nursing assistance, and limited respite for families caring for loved ones dying at home. Hospice can come into your home to offer limited services and also operates a number of facilities across the country where persons who need 24-hour care can go to die. The *National Hospice and Palliative Care Organization* estimates that the number of hospice patients nearly tripled between 1997 and 2006. In 2006, 1.3 million received hospice services and approximately 36 percent of all deaths in the U.S. that year were under the care of hospice (NHPCO 2007).

While most continue to die in the hospital, prior to death the majority of Americans live in home or community-based settings with the help of friends and family and occasionally home health services. Between 1992 and 1996, use of home health services rose, but in the wake of Medicare cutbacks, was on the decline again by the year 2000 (He, et al. 2005:66–7). In 2002, nearly 1.5 million Americans lived in nursing homes and the large majority of these residents were 85 or older (NCHS 2004). Nursing homes in the United States, however, are not created equal. Many nursing homes (typically those that accept Medicaid patients) are not places where you would want to be. Too often these places have the feel of a hospital, with white walls and easy to clean linoleum flooring. Residents may decorate their rooms a bit, but they do not typically bring in their own furniture and whatever efforts they do make do not seem to cut through the institutional feel. A walk through a typical American nursing home often reveals wheelchairs lining the hallways with residents slumped to one side, over-medicated and in various stages of consciousness or bedbound staring at the ceiling or the television in their rooms. If, however, you can afford to pay for long term care, the level of care and the atmosphere of the nursing home improve substantially. Assisted living is another, more recent option for persons who are elderly, require a minimum level of care, and can afford to pay for it. Having observed both systems from the inside, I find that certain nursing homes and many assisted living facilities that accept only private money (no Medicaid patients) in the United States are probably the closest comparison available to the majority of nursing home care that is available to all Dutch people.

Euthanasia and Assisted Dying in Cultural Perspective

We know that the Dutch and U.S. movements toward assisted dying originated from very different sources and ultimately took very different paths. The Dutch policy was originated by physicians frustrated with the kind of care they could give at the end of life in the face of life-prolonging technologies and treatments. In the U.S., assisted dying originated as a patient-led movement set, in part, in opposition to physicians and the medical establishment they represented. In The Netherlands, euthanasia became an option, preferred over physician-assisted suicide, which many Dutch physicians tend to think of as too messy and too risky. In the U.S., patients and families are largely left to their own devices or a patchwork system of end-of-life care and any talk tends to center around cost of care, withdrawal or withholding of care, and who has the right to make end-of-life decisions. Only occasionally does talk include assistance in dying in which the patient (not the doctor) takes his or her own life. In this section, I want to raise some potential explanations from a cultural perspective that could account for the differences in Dutch and American policies and practices at the end of life.

The Dutch Experience

Compared to the American experience with assisted dying, there are a few cultural practices that distinguish the Dutch experience with euthanasia and assisted suicide. In The Netherlands, there is a common practice of assimilating contradiction or conflict, there is an emphasis on making end of life orderly, and there is a unique relationship between citizen, society, and Nature that impacts end-of-life practices.

Dutch Assimilate Contradiction. The Dutch Golden Age is often attributed as the precursor for many current Dutch cultural traits and practices. During their 80 years war with Spain, The Netherlands formed their own nation. With the booming port cities of Amsterdam and Rotterdam, the Dutch rose to power in the 17th century as international traders, with conservative Calvinist views and a respect for artistic and intellectual freedom (Beenakker, et al. 1997; Mak 2000; Nijman 2000; Schama 1987; Zumthor 1994).[12]

British historian, Simon Schama (1987), characterizes The Netherlands of the 17th century as a culture based in contradiction. The rise of the Dutch nation, he says, was certainly founded on trade, but trade in the face of strongly Calvinistic views, creating a people balanced between abundance created by their mastery of trade and shame that came with the Calvinist emphasis on avoiding indulgences. Schama explains,

> As in so many other departments of Dutch culture, opposite impulses were harmoniously reconciled in practice. The incorrigible habits of material self-indulgence, and the spur of risky venture that were ingrained into the Dutch commercial economy themselves prompted all those warning clucks and solemn judgments from the appointed guardians of the old orthodoxy. It was their task to protect the Dutch from the consequences of their own economic success, just as it was the job of

---

12. The years of the Reformation saw the persecution of many great thinkers. The Netherlands rose as a free haven for those fleeing persecution in other European cities. Dutch historian Geert Mak writes, "[a]fter the toppling of the last medieval regents, the city [of Amsterdam] paradoxically grew into a realization of a medieval utopia: the safe, enclosed space in which the non-citizen could cast off the yoke of serfdom. 'This church consecrated to God knows not enforced beliefs, nor torture, nor death,' the Jewish immigrants, full of trust, wrote above the door of their Portuguese Synagogue. They called Amsterdam the Jerusalem of the West." See (Mak 2000, p. 108)

the people to make sure there was enough of a success in the first place to be protected from (Schama 1987:371).

Flexibility (and creativity) in the face of contradiction became key to cultural survival. Schama writes,

> The retaining membrane that held Dutch culture together for more than a century was a marvel of elasticity. Responding to appropriate external stimuli, it could expand or contract as the conditions of its survival altered. Under pressure, it could tighten to compress the Dutch into a sense of their indissoluble unity. In more expansive times it could relax and well, allowing for internal differentiation and the absorption of the whole gamut of beliefs, faiths, and even tongues (Schama 1987:596).

Today, The Netherlands remains a fairly open culture in the sense that as traders to Europe, they have maintained an openness to things foreign (foods, manners, and languages), which has the added benefit of easing trade relationships. But their openness is something beyond trade, it is a kind of cosmopolitanism, a pride in their ability as a small nation to be knowledgeable about things global (Lechner 2008). In the Chamber debates of 2001, Dutch political leaders demonstrate pride in their ability to be a melting pot of original ideas and social experimentation, embracing social policies that are often viewed as too radical for the rest of Europe. In the past, this meant offering refuge to the radical thinkers of their day. Today, it means offering refuge to such practices as smoking hash, engaging in prostitution, and assisting death.

An Orderly Dutch Process. Order and control seem to play an important role in the Dutch aesthetic. Cultural historian James Kennedy (2002) suggests that Dutch concern with euthanasia comes down to a matter of social control. The Dutch exert social control by making euthanasia *bespreekbaar* (debatable) in the public realm. By making euthanasia debatable publically, Kennedy says, the Dutch have imposed order on the hidden, taboo or otherwise chaotic by bringing these practices into the light of public scrutiny and debate (Kennedy 2002:16–18).

In private, euthanasia talk conforms to rules of Dutch *overleg*. *Overleg* is a very specific process of decision-making that is applied in many different realms of practice from deciding who in the workplace is responsible for cleaning the kitchen this week to deciding euthanasia policy on the floor of the First Chamber. *Overleg* is a process by which consensus-building occurs and decisions get made in politics, in business and in many other realms of social life in The Netherlands. Information is shared, superiors do not act superior, tempers and passions are kept in check, and in the end, a decision is made, diluted by compromise and majority rule. Van der Horst explains,

> The literal translation 'consultation' does not embrace the full meaning of the term in Dutch. [*Overleg*] is a form of group communication which aims not so much at reaching a decision as giving the parties involved the opportunity to exchange information. The Dutch spend many of their working hours in *overleg*. This means that they are discussing the state of affairs with their colleagues. They describe in detail the activities they are engaged in and the rest of the group are, in principle, entitled to make comments or ask questions (Horst 2001:170).

Van der Horst links a term, *gezelligheid* (which has no satisfying English equivalent) with the Dutch propensity for *overleg* (consultation). Van der Horst explains,

> [*Gezelligheid*] describes an atmosphere that the Dutch proudly believe is unique to them. The word itself is closely related to *gezelschap*, company. It is a form of behaviour, of communication, which keeps the people involved together because they appreciate it and it makes them feel good. *Ongezellig* behaviour on the part of one of the participants can ruin the atmosphere entirely. And the chance is always there because in a café or at a

party, it is no longer necessary to search for a consensus. People are there for fun. They can and do stand up
for their opinions. Controversial statements can be heard
from all corners. The danger then is that the *gezelligheid*
will be disrupted if someone does not permit another
to voice their opinions and attacks them personally
(Horst 2001:257–8).

To maintain *gezelligheid*, van der Horst suggests, people must be
heard and the process for deliberation must play out, thus *overleg*
relies more on the process of order making than it does on the end
result.

What the Dutch seem to favor is a process of decision-making
that is based on an aesthetic of order and control. Discussing something is quite different than acting on it and proper Dutch citizens
have choices, but that does not mean that they should act in ways
that communicate excess. The Dutch have a popular saying, "*Doe
maar gewoon, dan doe je al gek genoeg,*" which is translated to mean,
"Be normal, that is crazy enough" (Horst 2001:214). From the
Queen down to the prosperous businessman, Dutch citizens are
encouraged to downplay extravagance and individual achievement,
be it in wealth, dress or manner. They are encouraged to show re-
straint. This is not to say that Dutch people do not know extravagance. Any visitor to Amsterdam can see the wild side of Dutch life
played out by the orange-clad fans at an Ajax soccer match, in the
Amsterdam Canal Pride (a gay pride event along the *Prinsengracht*),
or in the wild streets of Amsterdam and other cities on Queen's
Day. As per their ability to embrace contradiction, typical Dutch citizens know when and how to demonstrate excess (Schama 1987:371).
Proper Dutch citizens are encouraged to conform to normative
standards that do not include overindulgence. Soft drugs are "legal"
in The Netherlands, but that does not mean that everyone should
smoke to excess. Euthanasia is "legal" in The Netherlands, but that
does not mean that everyone should die that way.

What the Dutch seem to be embracing in their euthanasia discussions is a process of making death orderly. The goal of euthanasia

talk, like any good example of *overleg,* is not about the end result. It is not about dying euthanasia deaths, but about living the remainder of your life in proper Dutch ways. Thus it is the process of euthanasia talk, not the final decision made, that creates the order for which Dutch people who participate in this discourse strive.

Dutch Faith in the Social Process. Some researchers suggest that the more radical social policies of the Dutch may have their origin in practices of tolerance (Horst 2001; Shetter 1987). One popular argument is that with over 16 million people on a piece of land approximately twice the size of New Jersey (CIA 2003), one-third of which was reclaimed from beneath the North and Zuider Seas, the Dutch have to be tolerant of each other's different views and needs in order to function and survive in such close proximity to each other and to the sea. This argument is embodied in the age-old image of the Dutch boy with his finger in the dyke. Everyone is responsible for the welfare of the town, thus even a small boy can save the town with just a finger in the dyke. A more recent version of this argument points to the fragmentation that occurred in Netherlands between the 1930s and mid-1960s. Dutch society fragmented into groups, or "pillars," based on shared ideology (Shetter 1987:178–183). People from the same religion or political affiliation had their own schools, sports clubs, unions, newspapers, radio and television programming. This required a policy of tolerance or a "compromise culture" to facilitate conflict resolution among competing concerns.

But can an ideology of tolerance alone account for such long-standing policies regulating prostitution, soft drugs, and euthanasia? Geographer, Jan Nijman, suggests that the concept of Dutch tolerance has perhaps run its course in The Netherlands, evolving into something that no longer resembles tolerance. Nijman explains,

> [t]olerance, perhaps Amsterdam's most prized commodity, is increasingly packaged and labeled to meet the demands of mass tourism and instant gratification. In the process it has become something of a perversion,

in the sense that it turned into a commercially motivated permissiveness that is in fact contrary to the city's
Calvinistic roots (Nijman 2000:41).

I argue that tolerance is not the best fit for what Dutch people do.
If the Dutch do not approve of something, they let you know quietly but unequivocally. It is quite powerful, for example, the social
reaction if you show up late for a meeting or speak out-of-line in
a social group. The line between what is done and not done is not
unclear. While many Dutch people seem to pride themselves on an
idea of tolerance, I would argue that the Dutch seem more committed
to order and process.

One of the more compelling explanations for euthanasia that I
encountered while in The Netherlands is the idea that the Dutch
willingness to control water (nature) is linked to their willingness
to control death (nature) by euthanasia policy (Rutenfrans 1997).
Many anthropologists have suggested that concepts of nature are heav-
ily impacted by cultural interpretation (Cronon 1996; Strathern
1992; Yanagisako and Delaney 1995). The Dutch relationship to
things natural is indeed unique. As far back as 500 B.C., the Dutch
were building *terpen* (earthen mounds) to hold the waters back
from their settlements and by the mid 20th century they had reclaimed one-third of their country from underneath the sea by a massive series of dykes, canals and polders.[13] I would argue that what

---

13. A polder, or section of man-made land, is created when dykes are
built surrounding a body of water. Windmills were then used to pump
out the water into canals that surrounded the polder. To keep the polder
dry, and inhabitable, windmills continued to pump excess water from the
polder. From 1927 to 1968, Dutch engineers drained large sections of the
Zuiderzee and other sections around the country resulting in one-third
more useable land. Over the years, there were periodic floods that destroyed large sections of land. The most recent was the flood of 1953 in
which 1,800 people lost their lives. The Dutch response was to engage in
the most ambitious project to date, the Delta Project. A large, moveable
dam designed to protect the southern delta regions from North Sea storms
(Meijer n.d.:6–17; Shetter 1987:31–39, 233).

began as an adversarial relationship with nature (when rains or high tides wore dykes away killing people and livestock and destroying land and homes), emerged as a relationship based on mutual respect and division of labor. The Dutch have a word that engineers use to refer to locks, bridges, tunnels and the like. The word is "*kunstwerk*," which also is used to refer to any "work of art." Shetter suggests that this word carries these two meanings not because the Dutch have difficulty distinguishing art from a bridge, but because to the Dutch "manmade modifications of [the] environment" are "works of art" (Shetter 1987:31). Nature provides Dutch people with raw materials (water, land, and Dutch life) and the Dutch shape these things to meet their needs (building bridges, reclaiming land from the sea, and orchestrating death). It seems little wonder that the Dutch are willing to help nature along in death. If they can make land, they can certainly (through talk of euthanasia) make death.

In The Netherlands, the beauty of nature is in the hands-on relationship that the Dutch have with it. It is what I would call an "aesthetic of co-construction" that is particular to the Dutch people; an aesthetic of existence that emphasizes human control in relation to natural boundaries and definitions (Foucault 1978). Schama argued that the Dutch perceive themselves to have Divine authority to co-construct existence. He explains,

> [T]he act of separating dry land from wet was laden with scriptural significance. 'The making of new land belongs to God alone,' wrote the great sixteenth-century hydraulic engineer Andries Vierlingh, '[b]ut He gives to some people the wit and the strength to do it.' In other words, the special favor of the Almighty had delegated to the Dutch a kind of license in the act of territorial creation (Schama 1987:35).

Today, nature, for many Dutch people, is no longer bounded by religion. In the 1970s, Europe experienced sharp rates of decline in church attendance and affiliation. The Netherlands, which had until this time been split between Calvinism and Catholicism, experienced some of the highest rates of secularization (Becker and Vink 1994). According to most recent figures, 42 percent of persons have no religious affiliation in The Netherlands, 29 percent are Roman Catholic, 19 percent are Dutch Reformed or Calvinist, and 10 percent represent other denominations (CBS 2008b). In a 2005 poll with participants from across Europe, the Directorate-General Research found that more Dutch respondents (27 percent) did not believe in God or a spirit/life force than any other country, with the exception of France (at 33 percent) and tied with Belgium (at 27 percent) (EBS 2005:9). The vacuum left by the rather abrupt move away from the Protestant and Catholic establishments may have provided many Dutch with the opportunity to replace God at the helm of nature. What was once a stronghold of Catholic and later Calvinist belief has become a nation that believes instead in the power of *their society* to take care of their own.

Just look at what the Dutch have done. They have reclaimed land from the sea. I once asked a Dutch water engineer if another flood (like the 1953 flood that killed 1,800 Dutch people and destroyed livestock, land and homes) was possible; not probable, but possible. *"Was het mogelijk?"* I asked. In the U.S., this would have almost been a blasphemous question. Of course floods are possible. It is nature and nature is unpredictable. You tempt it and it can even be wrathful. The Dutch answer was "no," a future flood that breaks through Dutch dykes is not possible. Why, I asked. The answer: because Dutch people have controlled for every contingency; they have it all worked out.

The combination of the Dutch relationship to nature and the hole left by secularization in The Netherlands has led to a belief—a faith—in Dutch society. Managing death by euthanasia is not a stretch for a society that believes itself to be on par with nature and with God. Euthanasia is simply an extension of what the Dutch already do with water and land. In euthanasia, the Dutch use what they are given by nature (the dying Dutch body) and they improve upon it, making death an orderly process that corresponds to their aesthetic of good and proper death.

The American Experience

The American experience is quite different from the Dutch. In the U.S., a Puritan ethic endures and the development of the individual in the context of distrust of state authority has led to a polarized view that juxtaposes the rights of the patient with the institution of medicine at the end of life. The U.S. system of healthcare is marked by a much more conflictive doctor-patient relationship, with threat of legal action that too often drives end-of-life decision-making and an aesthetic that favors individuals who fend for themselves over any type of comprehensive, state-supported system designed to offer assistance at the end of life.

Puritan Ethic. The Dutch have strong roots in Calvinism, which is often invoked as impacting the formation of their identity as a nation. The U.S. shares a strong identification with the Protestant movement, most notably Puritanism, in their formation as a nation, but in the U.S. that connection to religion endures in ways that it has not elsewhere. The U.S. was founded on religious freedom, populated initially by European adventurers, indentured servants, and those attempting to avoid religious persecution. During the Reformation in England, Protestants who did not conform to the Church of England were fined, whipped or jailed. By 1607, the first group of Puritans chose to leave England rather than face prosecution or conformity. These Pilgrims first moved to The Netherlands, then later returned to England to depart on the *Mayflower*, founding the Plymouth Colony in New England in 1620 (Gaustad 1990:51–5). These early settlers to the New World were Puritans whose beliefs centered on rejection of the authority of the church and elevation of the rights of the individual chosen. Boston clergyman, John Cotton, set forth the major complaints of the Puritan ethic at that time. According to religious historian Edwin Scott Gaustad,

> In the National Church, Cotton noted, the rule exercised by the bishops and the rigid conformity demanded by the law had become burdens too onerous to bear. The

use of the Book of Common Prayer, moreover, violated the Second Commandment which forbade men to bow down before the work of their own hands. Third, Cotton declared that the authority of the church should be congregational, not national; the highest human authority is neither king nor archbishop, but the members themselves. If that gave great power to the members, they for their part must prove themselves worthy of such power by giving evidence in their lives of their genuine conversion, of their having been chosen by God for eternal felicity with him. Finally, the church (said Cotton) is created not by legislative action from above, but by contractual agreement from below (Gaustad 1990:55).

The Puritan ethic laid the foundations for our nation, built on the rejection of both state and to some extent Church authority and a type of individualism that marked certain chosen individuals.

These religious overtones endure in the U.S. despite rhetoric about separation of church and state (Merelman 1984:1–26). When the rest of Europe was undergoing high rates of decline in church membership in the 1960s and '70s, the U.S. rates of church affiliation remained relatively constant. Compared to The Netherlands which has one of the highest rates of secularization in Europe, the U.S. has held relatively steady (Firebaugh and Harley 1991; Knippenberg 1998). In 2005, as many as 89 percent of Americans continue to identify with a religious affiliation (Bader, et al. 2005). As a result of this enduring connection, religion tends to frame our most heated public debates around abortion, homosexuality, and euthanasia. Compared to The Netherlands where the emphasis is on resolving conflict within Dutch parameters for public policy decision-making, in the U.S. conflict within debates tends to go unchecked. Many American debates on the end of life tend to get bogged down in polarized and often unresolved opposition between rhetoric around individual rights and moral and religious arguments of what constitutes personhood, family and proper ways to die.

Individual Rights vs. American Medicine. Much of the debate on end-of-life has been structured as an individual's right to make their own choices in the face of dominant systems of medicine and law. Not only are the way that people debate end-of-life polarized, but players within the debate (patients, families, physicians, medicine and the law) also tend to be in conflict. The American ideal emphasizes the individual, where individual's are encouraged to "pull themselves up by their own boot straps" and where the script of the American dream encourages the unknown and the unfortunate to achieve great riches, power or fame by their own devices. Where the Dutch favor the process of the collective, Americans tend to favor the rights of the individual to carve their own way. Our heroic stories typically portray the "Horatio Alger" persona who comes from nothing and through hard work, single-handedly achieves something great. We are a country that shies away from welfare programs and even those who support health care reform in the only industrial country without universal access must be careful not to represent reforms as "socialized medicine."

Political scientist, Richard Merelman (1991), studied some of the products of American culture including magazine advertisements, television sitcoms, and educational textbooks and found an American aesthetic that strikes a delicate balance between individual and institution. Merelman writes, "Americans represent themselves as flexible, impulsive, and egalitarian individuals willing to alter traditional roles, yet fearful of the freedom such alterations create" (Merelman 1991:102). Institutions hold power over individuals, limiting their choices and defining the playing field. The result is an American aesthetic that is neither fully individualistic nor fully democratic, leaving individuals somewhere between the poles of isolation and institutional domination.

In U.S. medicine, the patient-doctor-family relationship has often been viewed within medical anthropology as a relationship based in conflicting viewpoints, where the experience of illness and the means to return to health tend to be viewed in very different terms (Kleinman 1980a; Lock and Gordon 1988). The patient's rights movement which began in the 1970s for the first time in recent history threw the role of the doctor into question, originating from increasing criticism of psychiatry by Thomas Szasz, Erving Goffman and with such popular movies as, *One Flew Over the Cuckoo's Nest,* which exposed the institutionalization of mental patients as just another form of domination (Starr 1982:409). Where before physicians were popularly viewed to have the best interests of the patient at the forefront of their practice, the patients rights movement challenged both the balance of power in the doctor-patient-family relationship and the expertise of the physician (Starr 1982:389), opening the door for government regulation of medical practice and for medical malpractice claims by patients and families. Today, medical malpractice claims have steadily increased since the 1970s both in number and in the size of payouts (Budetti and Waters 2005; Thorpe 2004).

The cumulative effect is a health care system where insurance companies, the pharmaceutical industry and managed care meet in conflict with physicians and other health care professionals. Historically, the medical profession rose to power by restricting competition with other healers, by opposing legislation that would restrict their autonomy (including until recently opposing any efforts towards universal health care access), and by retaining authority to regulate themselves. Today, a shift is occurring. Rising health costs, an increasing supply of specialty physicians, increasing government and public regulation, and the rise to power of other industries such as the pharmaceutical, managed care and insurance industries are changing the way physicians do business. Solo and two-person practices like those that dominate Dutch general practice are no longer how most American general practitioners practice medicine. Instead, larger corporations are coming to dominate (Starr 1982:428–9).

This larger corporate system where the perspectives of the power players meet now dominates how medicine is practiced. Sharon Kaufman describes the result of this new system in her most recent book on death in the American hospital. Kaufman argues that death in the hospital is now marked by these pathways that no one entity has the power to stop. She writes,

Dying today is characterized by the making of choices among procedures. Things must be done. The pathways, the pressures to decide, and the language that defines the patient and rationalizes the timing of death are not freestanding entities. They cannot easily be removed or changed by individual actors or by institutional decree (Kaufman 2005:319).

This has resulted in an end-of-life system where some patients with no hope of recovery are receiving futile, costly and painful treatments that even health care professionals do not agree with, yet the system goes on.

Euthanasia in Historical and Cultural Perspective

In the Dutch Senate debates of April 2001, euthanasia was a rational decision made by a country bound less by religion than they are by a faith in society to take care of its own. Steeped in history and the Dutch familiar, euthanasia talk finds form. In The Netherlands, euthanasia law was the result of a largely physician-led movement, framed by physicians frustrated at the quality of care they could give at the end of life in the face of technologies and treatments that could prolong life but at a cost to quality of life. The debates give us some of the clues to the discourse on which euthanasia talk is based. Culminating from 30 years of public practice and debate, the Senate debates demonstrate which historical events were deemed relevant (e.g., Hitler Germany) and which were not (e.g., late Christian suicide taboos). The debates also gave hints to some of the main cultural forms that impact this end-of-life discourse, including the use of *overleg* (consultation) for assimilating conflict and dissent; an emphasis on order (e.g., *toetsing* commissions and reporting practices); and the unique relationship that exists between citizen, society, God and Nature.

Compared with the Dutch experience, the American experience is quite different and any attempts to bring aspects of this Dutch policy to the U.S. or elsewhere must consider precisely how these experiences may be historically and culturally different. In the U.S., a Puritan ethic has endured, placing the emphasis not on society to care for its own, but on individual citizens to care for themselves. In The Netherlands, the legal focus has been on physician's performing euthanasia for their patients, whereas in the U.S. the focus is on assisted dying, where patients make the choice to take their own lives. The American experience has been framed as a patient's rights movement, which sets patient and family interests in opposition to physicians and the medical establishment. It is based on a somewhat contentious doctor-patient-family relationship and without processes for managing conflict the movement for assisted dying in this country remains polarized and splintered.

PART II

Euthanasia Talk in The Netherlands

In 2001, approximately 34,700 requests for euthanasia were initiated with Dutch physicians, yet only 3,931 (2.8 percent of all deaths total) could be attributed to either euthanasia or assisted suicide. This means that approximately 1 in 10 of those who initiated a request for euthanasia with their physician (which includes those who initiated requests in the event of a future serious illness) died a euthanasia death and two-fifths of those who made 'concrete' requests (requests typically made after serious illness was diagnosed) died by euthanasia or assisted suicide. By 2005, less than 1 in 10 who initiated requests and only one-third who made concrete requests eventually died by euthanasia or assisted suicide (Wal, et al. 2003:46). With so many people in The Netherlands talking about euthanasia, yet so few going through with their request for euthanasia, it begs the question: what are Dutch people talking about when they talk euthanasia?

Euthanasia talk has emerged as a result of one prominent end-of-life discourse in The Netherlands. In the Foucauldian sense of the term, this discourse is a kind of script that shapes how many Dutch people have come to think, feel and act at the end of Dutch life. It is a script that encompasses end-of-life beliefs, fears, rituals, and norms. Euthanasia talk is deeply embedded in cultural practices that favor cooperation, dialogue, order, and faith in the efficacy of social process. Chapters 4, 5 and 6 are about the Dutch experience at the end-of-life and specifically their experience with euthanasia talk and euthanasia death. These chapters describe some of the experiences of euthanasia from the perspective of euthanasia talk's three most common participants: *huisartsen* (general practitioners), dying individuals, and their family members.

Where Foucault provides us with a framework for examining these experiences, Seale provides some options for understanding the content of euthanasia talk, suggesting that end-of-life practices may be a way of staving off social death. Social death can be defined as a series of losses that occur near the end of life that eventually culminate in a perceived disconnection from social life. Losses may be felt by the person dying or perceived by persons surrounding the dying individual. Social death is not absolute, however, and what one person may perceive as social death is not necessarily the same for another. Scheff (1990) suggests that there is an inherent drive people have to maintain sociality, to maintain a social identity and social relationships. Today, death most often does not happen in an instant, it is more typically a long process of life mixed in with decline and social losses that eventually (sometimes many years after an initial onset of terminal or serious illness) culminates in some combination of social and biological death (Lynn 2004:4–31). With so many people living longer and living with social losses and bodily decline, preventing social death becomes more important at the end of modern life.

Seale suggests that there are at least two ways that sociality is maintained at the end of life today. First, dying persons may transform social losses using a type of socio-therapeutic narrative that creates something meaningful and life affirming out of disconnection, decline and social loss. Second, dying persons may seek euthanasia or assisted suicide, to have the time of biological death (death of the body) adjusted to coincide more closely with social death (death of the social being) (Seale 1998:7–8). I suggest that what is occurring in The Netherlands at the end of life is something more complex. Dutch people are using euthanasia talk to bring concepts of ideal death to play in the everyday reality of bodily decline and social loss. In practice, euthanasia typically occurs as a discussion and not a life-ending act. Using euthanasia talk, many Dutch people are able to both create something meaningful in the face of social death and invoke a future ideal where biological and social death coincide to shape the production and interpretation of present-day reality. Euthanasia deaths when they occur allow biological death to occur more closely with social death, but in the majority of cases euthanasia occurs as a discussion that promotes ideals for Dutch social life and for Dutch deaths.

The following section uses data from a 15-month ethnographic study of euthanasia and end-of-life care in The Netherlands to demonstrate one country's response to social death in the modern era. Each chapter begins with an ethnographic story chosen to highlight many common themes from the larger sample of participants. Using these and other participant stories, I will show the reader one type of end-of-life discourse that has emerged in The Netherlands that provides many Dutch people with a script for the end-of-life based in Dutch ideals of life and death that gives participants some defense against social losses and bodily decline.

CHAPTER 4

A FAMILY FRIEND AT THE END: A *HUISARTS* PERSPECTIVE[1]

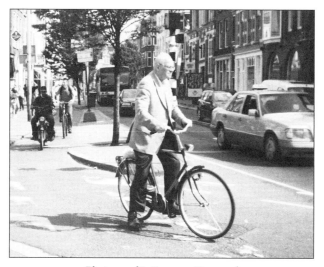

Photo credit: Frances Norwood

Huisartsen are gatekeepers to the Dutch health care system. According to the most recent figures *huisartsen* are responsible for approximately 87 percent of all euthanasia deaths that occur each year in The Netherlands (Onwuteaka-Philipsen, et al. 2007:102). Dutch general practice is unique and to understand how the majority of euthanasia deaths and discussions occur in The Netherlands, it is important to understand the *huisarts* practice. Fifteen months spent

---

1. Portions of this chapter were reprinted with permission by the editor of *Medische Antropologie* (Norwood 2006b).

with *huisartsen* in the greater Amsterdam region revealed that many considered their role at the end of life and, particularly in euthanasia talk, as something more than a typical doctor-patient relationship. One *huisarts* described it as a "fellow *lotgenoot* (companion in adventure or adversity) in the human condition of disease and mortality together with my patient." Many described the experience as a family friend doing a family favor. *Huisartsen* (literally translated to mean "house doctor" or "physician of the house or home") have a long and historically particular practice that seems to have eluded some of the larger global influences in medicine and general practice elsewhere. Somehow the Dutch have maintained an old-style, home-based practice in the midst of modern problems.[2]

This chapter is about the distinctive role of the Dutch *huisarts,* what they do at the end-of-life and what they think about their role in euthanasia. The chapter begins with an overview of Dutch general practice and a description of the Dutch *huisarts* that lays some of the groundwork for distinguishing key differences between Dutch and American general practice that may be impacting end-of-life discourse. Next, I will present an interview with one *huisarts,* a physician who spent some time contemplating what it means to perform euthanasia. Using his story and others, I will examine how *huisartsen* have come to interpret their role in euthanasia talk, how *huisartsen* are defining ideal death and invoking it in euthanasia talk, and finally how *huisartsen* may be facilitating social bonds and interpreting euthanasia discourse. Finally, I will talk about what happens when social bonds are not facilitated by *huisartsen* engaged in euthanasia talk.

---

2. This has not been easy to maintain, however. In the year I lived in Holland one of the most prevalent complaints by *huisartsen* was the increased volume of patients and workload. This, among other things, led to a call by the National *Huisarts* Association (*Landelijke Huisartsen Vereniging*) for a *huisartsen* strike in February 2001. While this strike did not go through, concerns by *huisartsen* remained eventually leading to a strike in May 2005 (VWS 2005).

A Different Kind of General Practice

Probably the single-most repeated mistake from both critics and supporters of Dutch euthanasia policy is the assumption that medical practice at home is equivalent to medical practice in The Netherlands. It is not. To understand euthanasia talk as a Dutch end-of-life discourse, you must first understand the unique nature of the *huisarts*-patient-family relationship. First, the setting of the Dutch *huisarts* is different. Dutch *huisartsen* tend to work alone in offices situated within neighborhoods, homes converted into office space typically, and they continue to this day a long tradition of conducting home visits, or house calls. In 1999 (the first year of my study), 77 percent of Dutch *huisartsen* worked either in solo practices or with only one other *huisarts*, although group practices are most recently on the rise (Griffiths, et al. 2008:20–21; Hingstman 1999:12). Rarely will you find a *huisarts* in an office building or other commercial setting. Eight of the ten *huisartsen* in my sample practiced in home-to-office converted settings, 80 percent were male, and at least half worked less than 40 hours per week. See Table 4.1.

Table 4.1 *Huisartsen* Characteristics,
Study Sample versus Population

Category	Subcategory	Sample Number (Percentage)	Population Percentage*
Sex	Male	8 (80%)	80%
	Female	2 (20%)	20%
Age	<40 years of age	1 (10%)	17%
	>40 years of age	9 (90%)	83%
Type of practice	Solo	3 (30%)	45%
	Duo	5 (50%)	32%
	Group (3 or more)	0 (0%)	14%
	Health Center	1 (10%)	9%
Time worked	Full-time	5 (50%)	70%
	Part-time	5 (50%)	30%

* *Source:* Hingstman, L. 1999. Cijfers uit de registratie van huisartsen. Utrecht: NIVEL.

Another important distinction between Dutch and American general practice is the power differential in the relationships between patients, families and *huisartsen*. First, unlike in the States where the relationship is more typically centered around the doctor-patient, in The Netherlands family members play a central role with the doctor-patient relationship throughout the life cycle. *Huisartsen*, particularly in smaller towns, typically treat the entire family and it is common for patients to be seen both at home and in the office with family members present. The power differential between doctor and patient-family is quite unique. In some ways, the power differential in terms of physician authority is more equalized between Dutch patients and *huisartsen* than between their U.S. counterparts, although I am told by *huisartsen* from other parts of the country that this varies by region. Dutch custom, in general, is to downplay difference in status (Horst 2001:23), and so doctors are encouraged to facilitate health, not proscribe it. Cultural historian Han van der Horst labels the practice an "engineer's mentality." He writes, "… many people and organizations see their tasks as largely a matter of stimulating or facilitating, promoting processes, guiding the activities of others" (Horst 2001:126). This is what Dutch *huisartsen* do.

This leads to the third most prominent feature of Dutch general practice, which is that the *huisarts* practice is largely a talk-based practice. Dutch general practice is based on dialogue with the patient and family members, providing information and building consensus. In a typical office visit, for example, the visit begins in the *spreekkamer* (or consultation room) seated across from or cattycorner to the *huisarts,* who is always dressed in regular clothing, no stethoscope around the neck nor white lab coat to distinguish roles. Most of the visit is spent seated around the physician's desk discussing the problem, including any psychosocial issues that the *huisarts* or patient deem relevant, such as stress on the job or problems in the marriage. Examination of the body always occurs second and sometimes not at all in a separate room called the *onderzoekskamer* (examination room).

In a typical morning of office visits, study *huisartsen* used the examination room in less than half (5 of 11) of all visits and the average length of a visit during morning office visits was approximately 12½ minutes, time usually spent in discussion. Afternoon office visits were often used to schedule patients whose health problems were more complex or psychosocial in nature. The length of afternoon visits varied more, some visits going as long as 20 to 30 minutes or longer and, like the morning visits, afternoon visits were typically based in discussion (Norwood 2005:164–168).

On the average, *huisartsen* in my study saw approximately 28 patients a day, which typically included at least seven house calls (Norwood 2005:164–168). House calls are generally conducted before lunch and at the end of the day and include visits to homes and nursing homes (*verzorgingshuizen*) both of which are domains of the *huisarts*. Every *huisarts* in my sample conducted house calls daily. See Table 4.2.

Table 4.2 *Huisartsen:* General Figures (n=10)*

Average length of office visit (morning)	12½ minutes
Average number of patients seen daily	Home visits: 7 Home/Office visits total: 28
Average number of patients (per practice) Percent of patients on *Ziekenfonds***	1828 62%
Total number of euthanasia deaths performed (2000–2001)	5
Cost of office visit (FY 2001) Cost of home visit (FY 2001)	fl 40,00 (=$17.10) fl 50,00 (=$21.38)

* Because of the small sample sizes, I do not assume that these figures are representative of population figures.

** *Ziekenfonds* was the former national health insurance program available to all Dutch citizens on a sliding scale fee and free of charge to those who not could afford it.

Compare that to a typical family practice in the U.S. American general practitioners usually work in office buildings, where the distance between doctor and patient tends to be well delineated. The American family doctor is dressed in a white lab coat with the stethoscope worn like a necklace to unambiguously communicate who is the doctor and what is most important, the examination. American patients meet their doctor often undressed, covered by a flimsy and uncomfortable paper gown in the examination room where any discussion typically centers on the examination. The doctor breezes into the room (there is not much time) and the patient has already been instructed by the nurse to remove any intrusive street clothing and to don the costume of the patient, the large paper gown. There is no time for discussion of home life or other psychosocial factors that may impact health and if that does happen, it is a short, perfunctory conversation that is only made more awkward when it occurs while a doctor is conducting the physical examination. Meeting in what the Dutch would call the *spreekkamer* to discuss health issues is not the norm, although there has been a trend with some doctors to start the first meeting with a patient in what the Dutch would call the *spreekkamer*, seated opposite a desk, clothes intact, to discuss generally why the patient has come. Also, the American *spreekkamer* is sometimes used after an examination when there are 'results' to communicate, particularly if they impact seriously on health. American family doctors do not have time, however, to discuss and no reason generally to include family or build consensus around everyday medical decisions. Factor in that most U.S. general practitioners do not conduct home visits and you have two systems that are in many respects quite different.

A Family Friend

In the course of my research, I spent much of my time with *huisartsen* in office visits and on house calls. One of the doctors I probably spent the most time with was Dr. Maarten Rohmer (not his real name). Even though we were quite different in personality, he was one of my favorite doctors, I think because both of us were drawn to how people experience end-of-life. Dr. Rohmer was soft spoken and older than many of the other *huisartsen* in my study, with a practice spanning almost three decades. Tall and good-looking with brown hair flecked gray at the temples, Dr. Rohmer was impressive in size, but quiet in demeanor. Dressed in the typical uniform of the Dutch *huisarts*, Dr. Rohmer usually wore jeans and a rumpled jacket with shoulders caved in from casual wear (no white lab coat for a Dutch general practitioner). Married with two grown children, he was a thoughtful man whose interest in euthanasia led him to explore the meaning euthanasia had for him both personally and professionally. The following is an excerpt of a taped interview in which we explored what it meant to him to talk about and perform euthanasia for his patients and his patient's families:

Frances: Why did you become a huisarts?

Dr. Rohmer: My father was a huisarts, *so he was an example for me from birth. I entered my studies, and, well, I don't like hospitals, from the inside they are dull and the atmosphere, I don't like. I saw so many fights against specialists and assistants and all those networks and they were angry, on the ground angry, and I don't like that as well. And I like continuity. I thought when I started to learn about being a* huisarts, *I thought that would be the most interesting thing, the continuity. You know people in normal, ordinary settings. I think that is one of the most important factors and as a specialist it is seldom that you know the whole story. I help with delivery and now the children that I delivered are having babies. That's the good part.*

Frances: Is your expectation of the importance of continuity turning out to be true?

Dr. Rohmer: Yes, and the longer I do it, the longer it is important, so I must continue.

Frances: What is your opinion about euthanasia?

Dr. Rohmer: Hmm [thinking], a good death with lots of possibilities. When all the circumstances are good, when it is well thought out initially and well discussed, not only between the patient and the doc-

tor, but also with the family involved, then it is a good death, a really beautiful death.[3] *It is beautiful to say your goodbyes together in a good form, in your own environment, then it is something you can look back on because it went well, that is a beautiful last day, a beautiful last day. If this always happens then it is a good death, but this doesn't always happen.*

Frances: Thus good communication is important?

Dr. Rohmer: Ja, for me euthanasia is really about communication, not only with folks who are dying but also with those who are intimately involved with the dying person and that is happening more and more. When I first did it that was not the most important aspect but that has grown to be more important. When I am busy with it I think more and more about the bystanders, about the people who remain behind and what it means for them. And if it is well discussed then it means also a peaceful death, a better death than at some deathbeds where things are not well discussed. That is important with euthanasia.

Frances: So is it what is left behind that is important?

Dr. Rohmer: Yes.

Frances: Because that is what is going to last a long time?

Dr. Rohmer: Ja, and people who have asked for euthanasia have assisted in this, they have been active and that is also important. A person can be busy with his future and that is much more clear-cut with euthanasia than with most deathbeds. Sometimes it happens naturally, of course, that people don't ask for euthanasia and that they are nonetheless well prepared with their family for the future, but with euthanasia that is more sharply defined.

---

3. Dr. Rohmer's exact words in Dutch were, "*dan is het een goede dood, echt een hele mooie dood.*" *Goed* translates fairly easily to mean "good," but *mooi* is a little more complex. The Van Dale definition of *mooi* includes 0.1 good-looking as in handsome, pretty, beautiful 0.2 lovely as in beautiful 0.3 smart 0.4 beautiful 0.5 good as in excellent 0.6 good as in fine, nice, handsome 0.7 good as in nice 0.8 pretty as in fine (Hannay and Schrama 1996:514). *Mooi* is used more in speech than *goed* and can apply to a much wider range of topics.

Frances: So you say that euthanasia is different from other deaths because in euthanasia more often you are talking about the future for the survivors?

Dr. Rohmer: Ja, *and that has possibly changed for me because I find that so important and that's where I begin but eventually the patient must deal with death within their own family because it doesn't end when you die, it goes on. Giving directives in death is so central that it brings the entire future into relief. Therein lies a clear difference than with other deaths.*

Frances: What exactly is the big difference between euthanasia and other deaths?

Dr. Rohmer: That someone who asks for euthanasia is forced much more than others to reflect.

Frances: Is euthanasia a natural death?

Dr. Rohmer: Not according to the law, but I find it quite natural. If euthanasia is a continuation of a medical condition then for me it is a natural death. It doesn't make so much difference, only a little extra push. The difference is not great enough to be unnatural.

Frances: You have been doing euthanasia a long time.

Dr. Rohmer: I have thought about it a lot. Why do I do it? A psychologist once helped me with that and he said, if someone is dying then the medical care is done, then it is more stepping back and maybe that is your strength. I am not such a doer. I am more someone who processes things, steps back and watches. I like to step back and perhaps guide them, but I am not someone who must wham-bam someone is sick and I must give them medicine and cure them immediately. No, I watch what happens. I am more a waiting person, that's what I am good at, I think. And if someone can't be treated anymore, then I still have a whole lot to offer: attention, warmth, but no medical intervention, no heroic measures. No treatment is sometimes better and I'm not scared to do that. I think that that is my personality — that I am not scared not to treat. That is what I'm good at. I notice with people who choose euthanasia or not that afterwards, after accompanying a deathbed, I am often thanked with presents.

Frances: If you're not afraid when the treatment has to end, there is nothing left to do in terms of the physical body, is euthanasia keeping you active as a doctor in the process?

Dr. Rohmer: I agree, more than without euthanasia. With euthanasia you can be active at any given moment and that keeps you pretty busy, while when there is no euthanasia, it's more hands off. I am more hands-off. When I know it's coming to an end, I don't need to go as often. Now, I go see patients frequently when it's near the end, but I don't need to. With euthanasia you have to do something. With that comes adrenaline, not only on the last day, but often before that. Each time I feel that talk is going in the direction of euthanasia, I become more awake, alert, active. It's really something different.

Frances: I wonder if that helps with that feeling of wanting continuity?

Dr. Rohmer: Yes, but that's not different with a natural deathbed. With a natural deathbed you still have the feeling that you finish things, but with euthanasia that is more exact, precise, more sharply defined. With euthanasia you are there at that moment that someone dies and with a natural deathbed you are called when it's over. Thus that makes it really personal, I finish it, the lifestory.[4]

Frances: But that is not the central thing?

Dr. Rohmer: No, but it's good to experience the deathbed, regardless of whether it's euthanasia or a natural death.[5] *It's important for me that I be there, maybe not at that exact moment but an hour or so later or a day later, and then again a week later.*

Frances: Is it a feeling of being needed?

Dr. Rohmer: Yes it's mutual, they need me and I need them. It really is mutual and that grows with almost everyone. There are only a few people where I think that feeling didn't occur. In my practice there

---

4. Dr. Rohmer's code switched between Dutch and English. His exact words were: "*dus dat maakt het heel persoonlijk, ik maak het af, the lifestory.*"

5. Even though Dr. Rohmer defines euthanasia earlier as a "natural" death, several times in our interview he makes the distinction between euthanasia and natural death (*natuurlijke dood*).

are a number of people I don't really get along with, some I don't really like, or don't have a connection with, but when it comes to the end, that relationship improves almost always.

Frances: And it doesn't matter if it's euthanasia or another form of dying?

Dr. Rohmer: No, that doesn't matter. It's about dying and euthanasia is a form of dying. It is one of the possibilities. The deathbed changes people, at least for people who need other people.

Dr. Rohmer's reflections touched me deeply and every time I re-read his words, I am struck by his ability to uncover and expose what is surely one of the more intimate relationships that occurs in life—helping someone else to die. His story brings up many important themes that I saw reflected in the stories of other *huisartsen* with whom I worked, three of which I will focus on in this chapter. First, I am interested in how Dr. Rohmer has come to think about his role at the end of Dutch life. He describes himself as someone who is comfortable not providing medical treatment at the end, yet he wants to be there when the person dies as both an observer/witness and as a more active participant in the dying process.

Second, I am interested in how Dr. Rohmer formulates "beautiful death" and how participation in euthanasia discussions facilitates his conception of ideal death. The elements of beautiful death that Dr. Rohmer raises were closely shared by other *huisartsen* in my study and appear to be impacting euthanasia talk and how Dutch people die. Third, I was struck by Dr. Rohmer's desire to deepen relationships with patients and families through participation in their death, especially in the case of euthanasia talk. The development and deepening of the relationship between *huisartsen* and families through the course of euthanasia talk was a theme that was raised repeatedly in the course of my research. The participation of *huisartsen* in euthanasia talk is not always conducive to maintaining social bonds, however, so I will spend some time exploring when this does not occur. In conclusion, I want to revisit the concept of the *huisarts* as a family friend to explore further how Dutch *huisartsen* have come to participate in Dutch end-of-life.

The *Huisarts* Role

The *huisarts* role in euthanasia talk fluctuates among a number of positions, from the more active role as guide to a more passive role as witness to something in between, a facilitator. When euthanasia is invoked it is a call to action and physicians in The Netherlands are clearly guides to that process. Euthanasia talk provides a framework and a structure for activities that occur at the end of life once euthanasia has been invoked. I have witnessed the shift that occurs when end-of-life discussions change to euthanasia discussions and it is literally as if a switch has been flipped. Once euthanasia is mentioned, the roles of patient, family and *huisarts* become more scripted (as Dr. Rohmer says, more defined) and a pattern of interaction emerges as several uniform stages of euthanasia talk begin (see also Chapter 2). Every *huisarts* with whom I worked, regardless of personality type or style, took charge of the euthanasia discussions. Verbal requests were discussed with the *huisarts* and with family members, and then had to be repeated by the patient in order to keep the process moving towards a euthanasia death. Written declarations for euthanasia were made and signed by the patient and (in all declarations that I saw) were signed by family members as well. If everyone was in agreement, then the process was typically paused until the patient was ready to move a request forward. If the request was re-initiated, then more discussions ensued with the *huisarts* leading the flow and the content of discussions with the patient and their family. In all cases, family members were included in discussions. If in these discussions, the patient clearly wanted to continue and there were no major reasons not to continue towards a euthanasia death, an appointment for a second opinion was made and then a date for euthanasia death was scheduled. In The Netherlands, patients may request euthanasia, but it is the physician's duty to decide whether a request meets the legal (and their personal) requirements for a proper euthanasia request.

What Dutch *huisartsen* do at the end-of-life is similar to what they do with any of their patients. Theirs is a practice that is based predominantly in discussion. Thus, it is understandable why Dr. Rohmer (and many other *huisartsen* in my sample) say that good death is about good communication and leaving good memories for family and other loved ones left behind. In fact, the *huisarts* focus on communication is even less surprising when you consider the broader social practice of *overleg* (consultation) that is prominent in Dutch social life.

Euthanasia talk and the roles participants assume in euthanasia talk follows rules for Dutch *overleg*. According to Dutch social historian Han van der Horst, *overleg* is "a form of group communication which aims not so much at reaching a decision as giving the parties involved the opportunity to exchange information" (Horst 2001:170). For proper *overleg* in the practice of euthanasia to occur, physicians must assume the role of facilitator and all participants (patients, family members, and physicians) must have the opportunity to voice their opinions and concerns. Patients will ultimately decide what they want, but they will do that in the context of a group process led by physicians with input and participation by everyone involved.

Every *huisarts* in my study told their patients to talk their request over with their family and every *huisarts* required that the patient speak repeatedly with family members and their *huisarts* about why they wanted euthanasia. In the end, most people did not die euthanasia deaths, but a lot of people talked about it. One Catholic *huisarts,* who agreed to talk about euthanasia with his patients but preferred not to perform euthanasia deaths if at all possible, argued that a patient's social environment (their friends and family) played the most important role in euthanasia talk. He said that patients naturally have anxiety and fear at the end, but if they can talk about their fears then euthanasia death is "almost never" necessary. He says, "It is normal to have angst [at the end of life]. But if you can go to someone and talk about what is bothering you, then often you can have a good life."

Finally, there is a witnessing aspect to what *huisartsen* do. Recall when Dr. Rohmer talked about his strengths as a *huisarts*. He said he had the ability to "step back" and "watch what happens." In a previous study of chaplains who minister to patients and families in a U.S. hospital, I found a similar practice that is in large part neglected in hospital medicine in the U.S., but does find presence in the work that chaplains do on the borders of hospital medicine (Norwood 2006a). I borrow the term, *witnessing*, from medical anthropologist Beverly Davenport who finds the term used by medical students in a homeless clinic to describe a practice that would typically not find place in mainstream medicine. It is a practice they described as "focus[ing] on the entirety of a person's life situation, not merely on their ailment" and as a way to "acknowledge the whole lives" of their patients (Davenport 2000:311, 316).

Dutch *huisartsen* take responsibility for end-of-life in ways that are not typical in the U.S. Dr. Rohmer tells us, "it's important for me that I be there," not necessarily to end life by euthanasia, but to be there to witness the passing of one of his patients, to be there for the patient and for the family. Another *huisarts* described the link between continuity and witnessing this way,

> The nice thing is the continuous care that you can give patients. You see people for many years and somebody you won't see them often and sometimes more often and some people get seriously ill and you have to guide them to the grave. When you just see a morning [of office visits] it's not so spectacular, but it's everything, the broad way that you see all types of diseases, minor to major diseases and you see them when they're so young and see them grow up, see them getting children and so on. Happy things and sad things, of course. That's the nicest thing, it's the continuous care.

Continuity and witnessing combine in such a way at the end of Dutch life, and most particularly in euthanasia talk, giving Dutch *huisartsen* a role that does not have a U.S. equivalent. *Huisartsen* are custodians at the end of Dutch life, serving in the event of euthanasia talk as both active participant and witness, from facilitator of discussions to a guide for patients and their families through the stages of euthanasia discussions. Their role as witness, though, is critical to ensuring that *huisartsen* do not get lost in activity at the end of life, activity that might push patients toward unnecessary treatments or unnecessary euthanasia deaths.

Making Death Beautiful: The Elements of Ideal Dutch Death

What made the prospect of a euthanasia death acceptable to all *huisartsen* with whom I worked, even those who performed euthanasia only in the rarest of occasions, was their shared belief that they were helping make death beautiful. I asked all study *huisartsen* to describe to me their version of an ideal case of euthanasia. Their answers were strikingly similar. When asked the first question about euthanasia, Dr. Rohmer replied that euthanasia was a "good death with lots of possibilities." Thus his first response was to invoke an ideal of what he thought all euthanasia cases should be. Good death, he explains is when the circumstances are good; it is well thought out and well discussed among patients, doctors and the family. Good death is peaceful and is conducted in a good environment (for most *huisartsen* this meant the home environment). Good death, Dr. Rohmer emphasized, is about communication and the memories that it leaves for survivors. Dr. Rohmer's conception of the good (the beautiful) death was quite similar to other doctors in my study. One *huisarts* said there was no 'ideal case for euthanasia.' The largest majority (5 of 10 *huisartsen*), however, said that an ideal case was well discussed; that there should be good family involvement; and that it was best when the patient did not have much longer to live and when the disease, like many forms of cancer for instance, was predictable enough to determine that. Three of ten *huisartsen* also described ideal elements that did not fit into a category. These included one doctor who liked to have the nurse involved in discussions and did not want to be rushed by the patient or family (a sentiment that was echoed by *huisartsen* in other research activities). Another doctor preferred to be involved in euthanasia and not assisted suicide because of the tendency of self-administered drugs to leave patients alive for hours or days (a sentiment that was echoed in other research activities). That same doctor also preferred the request to be a long-standing request for the purpose of ending physical suffering (a sentiment echoed during informal interviews with *huisartsen*). Still a third doctor preferred a euthanasia request for the purpose of relieving the kind of pain for which otherwise there is no relief.

Next, I asked what *huisartsen* thought the difference was between euthanasia and other deaths. What is it about euthanasia that helps or hinders good death? I asked Dr. Rohmer and he said that the patient's ability to give directives at the end, helping to create the memories that he or she leaves behind is quite different in euthanasia deaths. The Dutch words he used were "*dus de regie is zo centraal dat daardoor de hele toekomst ook in beeld komt, omdat hij zelf ermee bezig is en dat is een heel duidelijk verschil met het andere sterven.*" The word Dr. Rohmer used is '*regie,*' which invokes a theater metaphor. In Dutch '*regie*' means direction; production, as in the production of a play (Hannay and Schrama 1996:674). He said that when someone asks for euthanasia, they are also forced more than in other deaths to reflect on things. Having witnessed how euthanasia requests keep physicians active at the end of life, giving them a series of activities mostly based in discussion when otherwise most treatments have been discontinued, I asked if euthanasia kept him active in the process, feeding his interest in maintaining continuity in his patients' lives. Dr. Rohmer agreed that euthanasia requests kept him active in the process, but that did not necessarily mean taking action per se. For him, he wanted to be present often simply as a witness at the end of life and with euthanasia he found something "more exact, precise, more sharply defined" about his role.

Euthanasia talk offers a kind of script for ideal death, giving *huisartsen* a leading role in a process which appears to be more about affirming sociality than it is about funneling Dutch people toward early death by euthanasia. The numbers are clear. While a large number of people may enter euthanasia talks each year, only a few go through with it. In 2001 the year of my study, national figures indicate that of those who initiated a request for euthanasia with their physician (which includes those who initiate requests in the event of a future serious illness), only 1 in 10 died a euthanasia death and less than two-fifths of those who made "serious" requests (requests made after serious illness was diagnosed) died by euthanasia or assisted suicide. In 2001, euthanasia and assisted suicide accounted for approximately 2.8 percent of all deaths that occurred that year (Wal, et al. 2003:46). In my sample, 10 *huisartsen* performed a total of four euthanasia deaths and one assisted suicide death over the course of the study year. Over the course of their careers, study *huisartsen* performed euthanasia or assisted suicide on average only once every two to three years. And as you would expect, some *huisartsen* were more willing to perform euthanasia than others. One *huisarts* had only performed euthanasia twice in a 15 year career (see City2), while another had performed euthanasia on average a little more than once every two years of his career (see Town4). See Figure 4.1.

Ideal Dutch death certainly includes an element of control. Anthropologist Robert Pool (2000) examines the role of hospital physicians in a study he did on euthanasia in a Dutch hospital. Control,

Figure 4.1 Number of Euthanasia Deaths* Performed by Study *Huisartsen* (n=10) Compared to Years in Practice

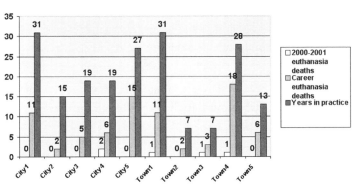

* Includes both euthanasia and assisted suicide deaths performed.

he argues, is the defining characteristic of the Dutch ideal of death, but how control is used in good and bad death is subtle. Suicide, for example, while it gives the person control to attempt death, is not a sure thing and a botched assisted suicide is usually not worth the risk for anyone involved (Pool 2000:212).

Assisted suicides typically occur with the *huisarts* present, but not active in the process. Because patients often are ingesting lethal drugs, vomiting may result making it difficult for the patient to ingest enough of the necessary drugs to ensure a quick (and orderly) death. Unlike euthanasia deaths, assisted suicide deaths often do not occur immediately. Sometimes the patient may fall into a coma for hours or days before dying and it is not uncommon for a botched assisted suicide to end in euthanasia death by lethal injection. For this reason assisted suicide is not considered ideal by Dutch standards. Assisted suicide, while just as 'legal' in The Netherlands, is rarely practiced. In 2001, approximately 0.2 percent of all deaths were the result of assisted suicide, compared to 2.6 percent of deaths by euthanasia (Wal, et al. 2003:46). I had *huisartsen* describe to me the difference between euthanasia and assisted suicide and many described assisted suicide (having a physician provide you with the means to kill yourself) as less predictable, less orderly and more drawn out than a euthanasia death. Only one *huisarts* expressed a preference for assisted suicide stating,

> I've never done a euthanasia. Both times I did assistance and it was a big relief for me to see that someone did it, that both patients did it themselves. It really made it much easier to accept.

Most *huisartsen* preferred to do euthanasia to cut down on the real possibility of a failed attempt. In the words of one *huisartsen,* "often enough [with an assisted suicide] the doctor still must give a *spuitje* (euthanasia injection) if the pills don't work." I asked study *huisartsen* if there might be a philosophical difference between assisting in someone's death and euthanasia and most, except for the *huisarts* quoted above, did not see a difference. According to one *huisarts,* both were done *samen* (together) with the family and the doctor.

The Dutch have a particular aesthetic about death that favors planning and regulation (rules and structures) over the unexpected or unplanned. Mystery or allowing 'nature' to take its course is not held in particular esteem in The Netherlands. It suggests to me that the long-standing relationship that Dutch people have holding the waters back, which has allowed as much as one-third of their country to be reclaimed from below the sea, has impacted how the Dutch have come to view death in its ideal form (see also Chapter 3). Dutch people control the water; why not also control death through talk of euthanasia?

Maintaining Dutch Families through Euthanasia Talk

Overleg at the end of life is not just a process for making decisions; I argue it is a manner in which Dutch relationships are defined. The emphasis in much of Dutch communication is on affirming a rather flat hierarchical social structure. Everyone should participate in *overleg*; and everyone should be able to communicate their perspective, but in ways that are conducive to consensus building, not counter to it. *Overleg* is a cultural form that gives shape to how many decisions are made in The Netherlands. To maintain *gezelligheid* (a warm, cozy Dutch atmosphere), a term that is invoked regularly in The Netherlands, people must participate in discussions, have their voice heard and be part of the process that guides the flow of Dutch life and Dutch decision-making.

There is a social element to euthanasia talk that encompasses two very important elements of the Dutch ideal that is evidenced in the *huisarts* role at the end of life. There is an element of social control, as touched on by Dr. Rohmer when he invokes the term '*regie*' (direction; production) and there is an element of social bonding and social affirmation that occurs during the course of euthanasia discussions. Euthanasia talk is an example of Foucauldian discourse (1972; 1991), where meanings of life and death are orchestrated and options for ideal death via one arm of society—the doctor — are managed. Euthanasia talk standardizes options for Dutch death, making an often uncertain and unpredictable time in life more certain and more directed. In the process, roles and relationships are affirmed through the patient-family-*huisarts* triad in the context of euthanasia talk (Seale 1998).

Dutch *huisartsen* assume a role at the end of life that does not exist in the U.S. It is a role that focuses on patient in the context of family and home. Euthanasia talk provides an avenue for *huisartsen* to assume an active role at the end of Dutch life, participating in the home and family life of patients and providing a structured space within home healthcare for participants to talk about and process meanings of life and death, and shifting identity in the face of social loss. U.S. healthcare is often criticized for leaving end-of-life patients in a no-man's-land once treatments are no longer needed (Kaufman 2005). In The Netherlands, dying individuals are typically not left alone to die. Compared to death in the U.S., those engaged in euthanasia talk in The Netherlands more typically spend their time as active, socially connected participants surrounded by an array of health and social supports. Their role in life may be diminished, but the structure of euthanasia talk holds them central.

In the beginning of my research, I was struck by the extent of the role that *huisartsen* assumed with the family, particularly once euthanasia was initiated. In the U.S., I would think that a general practitioner initiating a phone call to an estranged family member would be viewed (at the very least) as intrusive and (more likely) as illegal. This is not so in The Netherlands. At first, I thought that maybe this was a factor of living in a small town (where half of my sample was located), where everybody knows everyone else and *huisartsen* are often friends or social acquaintances with many of their patients outside of their practice. Comparison between my small town and Amsterdam study samples demonstrates that while city *huisartsen* have more transitory patient populations, more non-Dutch patients, and may have known their patients on average a shorter time, their orientation to their patients is similar to their small town counterparts. Small town and city *huisartsen* alike view their role in euthanasia discussions as a facilitator of family relationships.

Dr. Rohmer suggested that relationships with the family tended to deepen as a result of end-of-life practice. He says,

> Yes it's mutual, they need me and I need them. It really is mutual and that grows with almost everyone. There are only a few people where I think that feeling didn't occur. In my practice there are a number of people I don't really get along with, some I don't really like, or don't have a connection with, but when it comes to the end, that relationship improves almost always.

A number of *huisartsen* mentioned being thanked with gifts or flowers as a result of their participation in euthanasia death and every *huisarts* with whom I worked either mentioned or demonstrated that relationships tended to deepen in the course of euthanasia talk. When I asked another *huisarts* to describe a particularly satisfying occurrence of euthanasia, he says,

> Well, I can remember one from years ago it was a very old lady and it was physician [assisted suicide] and the sons and the family everybody was there at the house and she was just saying farewell to everybody as well as me. She kissed me and she said thank you and it was quite well, it was quite, I was just part, one of the family.

Still another *huisarts* says,

> When [the euthanasia] happened I found I had become part of the family. They all embraced me and thanked me for what I had done. In the church there was a service so I went there and in the service, the Quaker-like church, I was a kind of the guest of honor. It was very, yeah, it was very, I had not expected that.

Good death is not just about good discussions at the end of life, inclusion of family in euthanasia talk, or the image of family assembled around a deathbed. It is an emphasis on connection and sociality, on the bonds that keep Dutch people, even people who are dying, connected to Dutch society. Euthanasia death need not come to pass in order to achieve an ideal death scenario and while many end-of-life practices based in palliative care and general practice include the elements of fostering and maintaining relationships, it seems that in euthanasia talk, the roles are more clearly defined and a structure is in place that more clearly focuses on fostering bonds among participants. *Huisartsen* urge patients and their families to talk about the request (what it means and why) and in doing so, a linguistic space like what Seale describes is created for processing relationships, identity, and meaning at the end of life (Seale 1998:7–8). It is a space that allows dying individuals and families a place within home healthcare to re-work existing reality based on ideal constructions of a future where biological and social death coincide.

When *Huisartsen* Do Not Facilitate Ideal Death

A popular criticism of Dutch euthanasia practices is the 'slippery slope' argument, which suggests that allowing physicians to conduct legal euthanasia or assisted suicide would eventually lead to patients being killed against their will, particularly in vulnerable populations (Foley and Hendin 2002). All practices have limitations and there will always be gray (or liminal) areas where those limitations get worked out. In my study, I found that there are several ways in which ideal death and social bonds are not facilitated by *huisartsen* engaged in euthanasia talk.

First, according to Dutch euthanasia policy, *huisartsen* are given the daunting task of determining "lasting and unbearable suffering." The consequence of mandating such an impossible task is that sometimes they do it well and other times they do not. Current policy dictates, among other stipulations, that physicians must "hold the conviction that the request by the patient was voluntary and well-considered … that the patient's suffering was lasting and un-bearable … and that the patient holds the conviction that there was no other reasonable solution for the situation he was in" (The Act 2002). How is a *huisarts* going to meet these requirements, to determine what is 'voluntary,' 'well-considered,' 'lasting,' and 'unbear-able'? These are difficult concepts to operationalize in practice. Take the term 'unbearable,' *ondraaglijk* in Dutch. In euthanasia talk, *on-draaglijk* is typically invoked by the *huisarts* in response to initial re-quests for euthanasia. "Is your suffering *ondraaglijk?*" the *huisarts* asks. "Why? Why is it *ondraaglijk?*" The term comes from the *Ter-mination of Life on Request and Assisted Suicide (Review Procedures) Act* (2002). Quickly, the patient figures out that their suffering must be deemed "*ondraaglijk*" and so their answer, if they want to con-tinue is 'yes, it is *ondraaglijk*. But the pain, suffering, discomfort, and aches that go with dying do not translate well to measurement.

The *huisarts* response to these murky waters is often to invoke an ideal, to fall back on their concept of the ideal euthanasia patient and their ideal of what it means to assume the role of *huisarts* in Dutch society. Ideal *huisartsen* are concerned with the *whole* patient and input from the family. They are almost a family friend of sorts, re-sponding to ideal patients who have the right disease and know how to ask for euthanasia, how to suffer in proper Dutch ways, and who demonstrate the necessary connection to family and society. In euthanasia talk, the burden of determining "*ondraaglijk*" is ac-tually shared by patients, families and *huisartsen* structured within the discourse of euthanasia. Patients must be careful how they ask for euthanasia. Patients can wish no longer to live and suffer, but they cannot wish to die. Proper euthanasia requests are not suici-dal wishes. Depression and social isolation red flag the process, while predictable and definable diseases and disease trajectories make the process of considering someone's request for euthanasia less risky for the *huisarts*. Cancer, for example, is an ideal disease for "*ondraaglijk*" suffering, with predictable stages of decline and tan-gible symptoms of pain and discomfort. Illness due to old age and diseases of the heart, on the other hand, make the determination of *ondraaglijk* suffering much more difficult for the *huisarts*.

Falling back on constructions of the ideal (ideal disease, ideal patient, or ideal euthanasia discussion) and falling back on the shared process of decision-making (*overleg*) that is typical in The Netherlands, allows *huisartsen* some comfort in the gray areas of subjective determination in euthanasia cases. Gray areas persist, however, and it is inevitable that some people who "should" live by Dutch standards die and vice versa. Euthanasia law, for example, does not exclude emotional suffering and much of the public debates in recent years within The Netherlands have centered on where the limits of the euthanasia law should be in terms of what constitutes sufficient emotional suffering for euthanasia (NVVE 2000). Where does one draw the line between depression (not an acceptable reason for euthanasia) and "lasting and unbearable" emotional suffering (an acceptable reason for euthanasia)? At the same time, certain people come to be excluded from engaging in euthanasia talk that might benefit from it. In my study, I found that aging and being elderly is not necessarily a reason to die and newer immigrants, not versed in Dutch ways of engaging in this discourse, are often turned away from euthanasia discussions.

Another way in which ideal Dutch death is not achieved is when *huisartsen* end life without following proper euthanasia procedures. One *huisartsen* with whom I spoke told me about a patient who was in his 80s who was seemingly healthy and active until a heart attack landed him in the hospital. Once there, it was discovered that he had inoperable, end-stage cancer. According to his physicians, he had only a few days or a week left to live. They brought him home to die and the family asked the *huisarts* to "*hem te laten inslapen*" (to "let him sleep"). They said it was what he would have wanted. The *huisarts,* who knew the man and his family well, told me that he had spoken to the man and his wife before he fell ill at which time the man had "made his wishes clear." If the time came, he would not want to die hooked up to machines and would want assistance in dying. The *huisarts* held a meeting with the family and once it was established that they were all in agreement that this was not the way he would have wanted to live, the *huisarts* increased his morphine with the intention of addressing pain and unrest, but with the "first priority" to hasten death. The man died two days after coming home from the hospital and three days after life-sustaining nutrition was removed. The *huisarts'* behavior was legal in The Netherlands, falling under a category of "normal medical practice" in which increasing medication for pain relief is acceptable, regardless of the doctor's subjective intention to hasten death. This particular practice is called, "terminal sedation." Terminal sedation is a type of medical behavior that potentially shortens life (MBPSL) due to sedation accompanied by withholding of artificial nutrition or hydration for a period long enough that it can be expected to hasten death (Griffiths, et al. 2008:64–66). While this case is technically legal and represented the previous expressed wishes of the patient, it is a type of MBPSL that is in need of further discussion and regulation so as not to serve as an unregulated alternative to euthanasia in The Netherlands.

A Friend of the Dutch Family and an Agent of the State

Huisartsen described what they do at the end of Dutch life akin to a family friend doing a family favor. In the course of euthanasia talk, Dr. Rohmer and others said the bond with patients and families typically grew stronger and it was not unusual to receive thank yous or gifts, such as flowers, in the aftermath of euthanasia talks. There is more to it, however, because the *huisartsen* is situated between several competing concerns—the concerns of the profession versus the concerns of the family, concerns of his or her personal beliefs versus the concerns of the state. The *huisarts'* role as family friend is not sufficient to describe what they do, because *huisartsen* really are not family and must act in accordance with their own personal beliefs, professional ethics, state policies and shared cultural understandings. *Huisartsen* in euthanasia talk are themselves guided by a discourse that has emerged to give them assistance and direction for managing Dutch death.

Euthanasia is a burden that *huisartsen* and other doctors in The Netherlands carry, but they do not carry it alone. The Dutch are a consensus-building society and no burden is carried by one member alone; it is shared. The Dutch system has been criticized for rarely punishing doctors who do not follow proper euthanasia procedures (Griffiths, et al. 1998:43–85). According to recent figures, Dutch prosecutors gave only 13 indictments in euthanasia cases over the course of 15 years of legal practice and some 7000 reported cases (Griffiths, et al. 2008:138). Legal control over euthanasia and assisted suicide in The Netherlands relies on self-reporting by physicians (Griffiths, et al. 2008:126). According to the Law on Burial and Cremation, physicians must file a death certificate certifying whether the patient died of "natural" (e.g., disease related) or "non-natural" causes (e.g. euthanasia or assisted suicide). Prior to 1998, there existed a number of ways that a "non-natural" death could reach prosecution. By 1998, regional review committees were established to assess physician reports of "non-natural" death. Once a physician fills out a death certificate certifying "non-natural" death that information is examined by the coroner and then sent to a *toetsingscommissie* (regional review committee), along with medical notes from both the treating and second opinion physician and the patient's medical file. Between 1998 and the introduction of the *Termination of Life on Request and Assisted Suicide (Review Procedures) Act* (2002), review committees had the power to advise the prosecutorial authorities on whether or not the physician's actions met Requirements for Due Care established by the Royal Dutch Society for the Promotion of Health, formerly the Royal Dutch Medical Association (KNMG). After 2002, the new law established the power of review committees to be the final decision about whether or not a case will go to prosecution. As of 2008, however, no case determined by regional review committees to be "not careful" has been prosecuted (Griffiths, et al. 2008:128, 214–15).

If doctors are not being punished for indiscretions in euthanasia practice, then, ultimately, they are not the ones being held accountable. Dutch law was reached by countless years of cultural practice and by more than 30 years of public debate and consensus building. Dutch *society* created the policy and the state (through its policy) manages the burden of life and death, yet who is accountable is less than clear.

Dutch huisartsen are situated somewhere between the Dutch family and the Dutch state. One *huisarts* described the precariousness of this position as falling somewhere between a 'hero' and a 'criminal.' I have observed first-hand the reporting procedure on the day of a euthanasia death. Typically prior to death, the *huisarts* contacts the local coroner who comes to view the body after death, determining that death has occurred and to review the documentation provided by the *huisarts* in the case of a "non-natural" death. The coroner and the *huisarts* meet to discuss any questions related to the documentation and the coroner leaves, eventually forwarding the paperwork to the regional review committee. *Huisartsen* tell me that waiting to hear from the committee feels like a criminal waiting for a verdict. I have been in the office when a *huisarts* takes the phone call from a review committee member, relieving them from the threat of prosecution. The tension, even when the case is nothing unusual, is high. To the family and the patient, however, the *huisarts* is often viewed as a type of hero—the one member of society who is willing to stay with them through to the end of life, letting them know that society will not abandon them, eliciting talk and planning for ideal death, witnessing the end of the life, and occasionally stepping in to actively end life.

Given the daunting task of managing end-of-life and (when deemed appropriate, ending life through euthanasia death), *huisartsen* in The Netherlands have learned to use euthanasia to provide their patients and their patient's families with a death that approximates an ideal. They do this by means of an ideal script (euthanasia talk) that helps participants at the end of life bind and re-formulate concepts of self and society, identity and relationships disrupted by bodily decline and social losses. *Huisartsen* also approximate ideal death by means of an act, either invoking an ideal future act to help shape the interpretation of present reality or in a few cases allowing biological death to more closely coincide with social death by euthanasia.

CHAPTER 5

INTO THE GARDEN: EUTHANASIA TALK AND THE DYING INDIVIDUAL

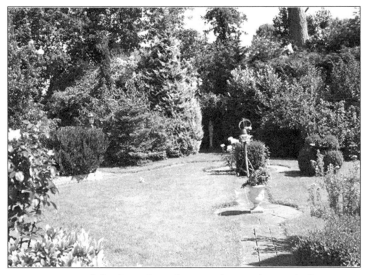

A Dutch back garden. Photo credit: Nicole Marshall

Dutch people have a special connection to their gardens and during my stay in The Netherlands, I came to see the garden as one expression of Dutch individuality. Many Dutch homes and ground floor apartments have a backyard garden with a 6 to 8 foot fence typically high enough to keep the eyes — but not the ears — of the neighbors at bay. With the premium on space in The Netherlands, gardens are small, but packed with personality. A few are tended to give the impression of nature in the wild, many others, however, are more controlled, more sculpted — showcasing exotic plants, tiny walkways and benches nestled among neatly manicured rows of flowers and plants. Visitors to 17th century Holland also noted the unique status that Dutch gardens held. According to architectural historian, Wytold Rybczynski, "the Dutch prized three things above all else: first their children, second their homes, and third their gardens" (Rybczynski 1986:60). Dutch gardens were different from other European gardens, which tended to be public spaces, shared by several townhouses. The introduction of the Dutch garden coincided with the shift from a communal big house to individual family homes in The Netherlands and these gardens were constructed to be private and orderly spaces with "precisely clipped hedges, geometrically shaped box trees, and colored gravel walks [echoing] the orderliness of the interiors" (Rybczynski 1986:60).

Today, Dutch people continue to prize the back garden. Gardens are a status symbol and when Dutch people talk gardens, they talk about the size of the garden (slightly larger is better) and how well kept it is. As Han van der Horst emphasizes, gardens "must be as strictly controlled as possible" (Horst 2001:115). An overgrown garden is akin to a dirty front stoop or dirty window panes; it is not the sign of proper Dutch living (Horst 2001:115, 245–249). I mention the Dutch garden because it was something that figured prominently at the end of Dutch life. Many who were sick or dying at home (and who lived on the coveted ground floor), typically placed their bed in the living room next to the large picture window that overlooked the back garden. Having spent time as a hospice volunteer in the United States, I cannot help but to compare that with the more typical scene in American homes, in which the dying individual is often situated in front of a television screen that is rarely ever turned off. Watching television is not how most Dutch people (living or dying) spend their time.

This chapter explores what it means to engage in euthanasia talk from the perspective of dying individuals. I want to describe what it feels like to experience life at the end of life and I will examine some of the consequences of dying and how euthanasia talk impacts that experience. I will explore the role of the dying individual in euthanasia discussions and how these individuals interact with family and *huisartsen*. I will explore how euthanasia talk keeps people connected to family and society and I will explore when it does not. Finally, I want to talk about what is distinctly Dutch about this way of dying and what it means to want to die overlooking your own garden.

The chapter begins with the story of a gay man who was diagnosed with HIV in the mid-eighties. A month before I met him, he came very close to dying due to complications from AIDS. When we met, he had a euthanasia request in writing with his *huisarts* and had had multiple conversations with his *huisarts*, his partner and his family about his request. This is the story of what it was like to come so close to death and why he chose to initiate a request for euthanasia.

Into the Garden

I met Matthijs [pronounced Ma-TAYS] and his American partner, David, on a cold, clear day in February 2001. They live not far from the center of Amsterdam in a Dutch flat on the coveted ground floor. (Unlike the other apartments in a multi-story building, only ground floor apartments have the desired private garden in the back). It is a typical city apartment with small, narrow rooms and large, bare picture windows overlooking the street in the front and the garden in the back. David and Matthijs welcomed me and after settling in the living room over tea and cigarettes, we began what would become a series of intense discussions about life and death, love, religion, and the differences between Dutch and American societies.

I took to them both immediately. David, the more boisterous of the two, is an American man, cute and boyish looking in his mid-forties. He is the kind of guy I love to be around, the kind of guy who talks with his hands and marks his speech with big theatrical pauses and expansive looks that bring everyone around into his conversation. Matthijs, tall with the Dutch angular jaw and dark curls around his face, clearly loved David's outgoing style, complimenting it with his own quiet, yet thoughtful responses. I asked how they met and David told me they met at a sauna in the early 1990s. A week later, they were sitting around David's apartment after dinner and a movie, and Matthijs dropped that he would probably die before his mother. David, who had already lost one partner to AIDS, picked up on that, asking outright, "Are you HIV+?" Matthijs replied, "Yes." David reacted immediately, jumping up from his seat to go over and put his arms around Matthijs. "It just makes me love you all the more," he said hugging him. "We've been together ever since," David tells me, with a long sideways glance at Matthijs who had obviously heard this story before.

Matthijs was diagnosed with HIV in 1986 when he initiated an HIV test because "everyone else was getting one." The results were wholly unexpected and he remembered reflecting on how healthy he felt at the time. He remained asymptomatic until 1994, when he had minor health complications. In 1996, he started with protease inhibitors even though he was not sick. I asked why and he said they were popular at the time, touted as the miracle cure, he said. Matthijs experienced serious liver problems in 1997 and more complications in 1999. By summer 2000, Matthijs found he was resistant to many of the protease inhibitor combinations and stopped taking them.

AIDS dementia was the next health scare, complicated by a long lag time in diagnosis. For David, a former nurse in the United States, this was just one of a long series of frustrations with what he described as the sluggish and at times non-responsive Dutch medical system. By January 2001, Matthijs was so ill that he and his doctors believed that he had only days or weeks to live. He rallied, however, and fueled by David's willingness to question the system and against his family's wishes, Matthijs stopped all medical treatments in February 2001. Now, he tells me, he doesn't want to know whether his viral lode is high or his T-cell count is low; he just wants to live the life he has left.

Matthijs has a euthanasia request on file with his huisarts, *Dr. de Boers, and has continued to maintain somewhat of a relationship with her even though he has stopped all treatment with his specialists. I asked Matthijs and David whether they had talked the request over with Dr. de Boers and they said they had. They had several discussions with her and both came away feeling that Dr. de Boers would help them at the end if they needed it. This is what they had to say:*

David: She couldn't promise me that he wouldn't have pain, but you know if she had said that I wouldn't have believed her. She said she would do her best to make sure he didn't suffer unnecessary pain. She said when there are breathing problems, for example, it is often more difficult for the family than it is for the individual. It is traumatic to watch. But she can come here four times a day if it's necessary, as much for the family as for Matthijs. I've had so many difficult experiences with the doctors here. The first couple of times I spoke with Dr. de Boer, I had the impression that she didn't want to listen to me. After that I took her aside and made it clear how important it was for me that she be direct but also sensitive to where I was coming from. Now I know that I can say what I want to her and that [we're clear].

Frances: And for you [Matthijs] how did that decision come about?

Matthijs: Well [big pause], I always felt, I'm not afraid of dying, but of dying worried. I've seen both my parents die and in their cases there was no ... They were ... The whole idea of euthanasia was abhorrent to them but what happened by the time they couldn't really breathe anymore, they got a shot of morphine. And of course it wasn't euthanasia, and yet the effect is more or less the same.

Frances: It did end their life?

Matthijs: It did end their life within 10 minutes of the shot, but of course you can't go by the government definition of euthanasia because they'll get upset. "Of course, I don't do that." I was talking about it with Dr. de Boer when I was trying to figure out my feelings about euthanasia. She said, "I've done euthanasia, but I'd rather not." [and I told her what had happened to my parents and] she said "no, no, no, that is NOT euthanasia. That's not what we're talking about." But to me it comes down to the same thing, except in my case, I don't know how to say ... some people say, "Ik ben zo benauwd[1] (I am so anx-

---

1. *Benauwdheid* is used by patients and physicians to describe a symptom that has both physical and mental attributes. It is translated to mean "tightness of the chest," "closeness, stuffiness," "fear, anxiety," and "distress" (Hannay and Schrama 1996:81). In end-of-life care, it signals an

ious/I have tightness in my chest)" or somebody else says, "Hij is zo benauwd, is er iets tegen benauwdheid, dokter? (He has anxiety/tightness in his chest, is there something for [that], doctor?)." Ja, as long as you don't call it euthanasia.

Frances: Was the purpose to shorten their life?

Matthijs: No, it was for the pain. At the end, [my father] asked for a spuitje[2] *for* benauwdheid. *And noone spoke about euthanasia or ending life. Not the doctor. Is it euthanasia or is it palliative care?*

David: And without oxygen for benauwdheid *your brain doesn't get enough oxygen and then you're confused. I am against euthanasia myself. It's difficult to get euthanasia here. Dr. de Boers was [like] whoa when we talked to her about euthanasia. And I thought, you come to Holland, you want a* spuitje *and boom there it is.*

David and Matthijs: [at the same time] Totally not the case.

At this point in the conversation, David who was already late for an appointment had to leave, but he and Matthijs suggested that I stay a little longer. We continued our interview.

Frances: So why euthanasia?

Matthijs: I'd rather die, uh, but if you can't control your future and another factor is because David's other partner suffered quite badly and it was a real strain on him. It was made worse because the doctor [at that time] advised not to let the patient know it was a terminal situation.

Frances: What did David's last partner die of?

Matthijs: AIDS.

Frances: But they didn't know that it was terminal?

Matthijs: Everybody around him knew, but he didn't. He didn't know. He knew that he had AIDS, but only they knew that he was dying.

Frances: Was this in the U.S. or here?

Matthijs: That was in the U.S. And David was quite young and it was a real situation. Especially at the end when he was losing his mind

acceptable term of suffering that can warrant an increase in morphine. Its use marks one of the liminal areas in euthanasia and end-of-life care.

2. Asking for a "*spuitje*" (syringe), is one typical way patients may ask for euthanasia. "*Ik wil een spuitje*" (I want a syringe).

and obviously in a lot of pain and there was no help. To take the anxiety away I wanted to have a euthanasieverklaring *(written euthanasia declaration). Although for euthanasia, this is just a piece of paper, it states what you want but it doesn't have much [pause]—you don't have any right to euthanasia when you give them this. And we had a couple of negotiations with Dr. de Boer about her euthanasia attitude, so at the moment we feel, how would you say, optimistic? Good?*

Frances: So she has agreed that she will do it for you if it is necessary.

Matthijs: [She has agreed] that she is not opposed to it per se—to be here, to perform the procedure. Which I think is a good thing. I talked to some other doctors before who were easy about it, but [that] didn't make me feel comfortable. Like they would say, "Yeah, no problem at all. No problem at all. It's so far, so you just tell me." I think when it's that easy I don't really trust it. Because, ja, *when you are in the medical profession, basically you want to keep people alive. In some situations it's nearly impossible to save somebody and I'm sure for the doctor that must be a really frustrating and pressing thing to perform a euthanasia, because otherwise, you wouldn't have wanted to become a doctor. So I feel pretty [content] with Dr. de Boer, but I do hope when the time comes that I'll either die in my sleep or die staring outside into the garden. We don't know. The way my parents died. They were sick and got sicker and that's how I might die. When I was really sick I was thinking a lot about something, at the moment, I was really … When you get sick you feel different about a lot of things. You get much more emotional, less rational; not just about your own life, but about relationships as well. [phone interruption]*

Frances: You were talking about what you think when you are feeling sick.

Matthijs: Oh [pause]. Like you want to make up stuff. You realize you don't want any bad feelings anymore … Feelings become so important. When you start feeling better, you kind of get back to your old self.

Frances: Is that good [laughing]?

Matthijs: On the one hand yes, on the other hand, no. I had the kind of education where you don't show those kinds of emotions, men don't cry, that kind of thing. When I felt that I was dying, I didn't mind about crying or being emotional or making a fool of myself. Those kinds of things I don't remember anymore ... I hadn't expected that the feeling would go away with the return of my health. But it is logical, of course, a lifetime of conditioning. That doesn't leave you all of the sudden.

Frances: What kind of treatment do you want to have at the end of your life?

Matthijs: For me, I have no need for medical interventions to remain living.

Frances: Do you have a living will that states that?

Matthijs: Ja.

Frances: And your plan is to stay home or will you go to the hospital if you need to?

Matthijs: Under no circumstances do I want to die in the hospital. I hate hospitals. You have no privacy. And you have no control over when to sleep and when to bathe.

Frances: It's too regulated?

Matthijs: Ja, it's regulated and you are totally powerless. You lie in a ward with all these people, but of course when you're dying you get your own room, but even then it is strange. I don't know if you've ever been laid up in a hospital. It's not comfortable. The mattress and the pillows are plastic with only a sheet over them. At home you have your comfortable bed and down-filled pillows. When you sweat in a hospital bed, it's terrible. [Everything is wet]. At home, you're in your own surroundings; you have your cat and your partner, but I do understand it is a luxury to want to die at home. And at home you do have to be dependent on someone to care for you.

Frances: If you could paint an ideal picture, what kind of care would you want to have?

Matthijs: That is a difficult question to answer. In my ideal world no one would get sick and no one would die. But preferably, ja, the ideal care is the kind of care that you receive from your mother, who is constantly around and always ready to help. In that regard I've been very lucky. You can't always control whether you will have a partner in your life or not. And I don't think I'd still be here if I was alone in the world. Alone? Naturally you always have friends and family, but someone who really cares for you. Cares for you in practical and material ways, but also in spiritual ways as well, someone you can go deep with. I've been really sick a few times and few times I came to the point where I thought, if I wanted, I could let my life slip away. But if there is a reason to go another day, then I could do that too. I think when you have someone who cares for you and loves you, then you can say I want to go another day or another week. Which gives me the idea, my ideal situation would be to stay healthy, to be able to remain standing seven hours a day, and to go to work. Then I could complain about that instead.

Matthijs' story is a little different than some that I heard and witnessed while in The Netherlands. First, he was the only person with whom I worked who had HIV. While ten years ago HIV and cancer made up the majority of euthanasia cases in The Netherlands, changes in the efficacy of AIDS treatments seem to have brought about a sharp decline in the number of persons with euthanasia requests dying of AIDS related illnesses (Pool 2000:241; Wal, et al. 2003:49).[3] He was also one of the few who had come to the brink of death and returned able to express to me in words what it felt like to experience dying. Matthijs' story is in many ways, however, similar to the other stories that I heard and experienced in The Netherlands. His story (and theirs) reflect common themes. In the following sections, I will focus on how euthanasia talk is used: (1) as an ideal scenario that empowers individuals who are dying and provides them with an emotional insurance plan for the future and a venue for processing what it means to die; (2) as a mechanism for exerting control and order in the face of bodily disruption; and (3) as a mechanism for staying connected with family and society at the end of Dutch life.

---

3. In 2001, 77 percent of all euthanasia cases were persons with cancer. Four percent had heart or blood diseases, 4 percent had diseases of the nervous system, 5 percent had lung diseases, and 10 percent had other illnesses that were life threatening (Wal, et al. 2003:49).

Making Death Ideal

Matthijs alludes to an ideal throughout his interview. At one point Matthijs talks about his request for euthanasia and says he was content in knowing it was an option, but his hope was to die in his sleep or staring out into his garden. He followed that with the description of his parents' deaths, how they got sicker and sicker, until they couldn't breathe anymore. He described their deaths as messy and disorderly, eased only by increases in morphine, which finally was used to purposefully hasten both of their deaths. For Matthijs, ideal care at the end of life is like that unconditional care that you get from your mother, surrounded by family and the comforts of home. He, like many of those I met who were dying, did not like the hospital, which according to Matthijs was too *geregeld* (regulated), often uncomfortable, and rendered him feeling powerless. Looking at the larger sample of those who were dying, the Dutch ideal is to die at home, surrounded by loved ones, and without too much pain or suffering.

Home vs. the Hospital. Matthijs came close to dying in a hospital a month before I met him. That and many other hospital experiences made him adamant that he did not want to die in the hospital. In the hospital he felt separated from the comforts of home, his own bed and his family. He was surrounded by strangers and felt that regulations about when to bathe and when to eat rendered him powerless, a thought expressed by many who have encountered hospitals, not just in Holland (Glaser and Strauss 1968; Kaufman 2005; Pool 2000; Puchalski 2006). One study participant says, "we're getting attention now that we're out of the hospital," suggesting to me that the *kind* of attention that one receives in the hospital may very well be qualitatively different than the kind received at home, through the *huisarts*.

In my sample, 17 of 25 patients with whom I conducted intensive case studies chose to die at home, seven lived in nursing homes (*verzorgingscentra*), and one lived in an acute care nursing facility (*verpleeghuis*). See Figure 5.1. Since the hospital was the one end-

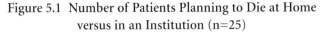

Figure 5.1 Number of Patients Planning to Die at Home
versus in an Institution (n=25)

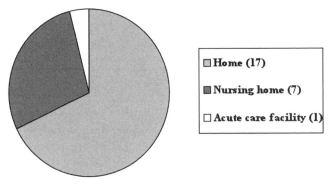

☐ Home (17)

■ Nursing home (7)

☐ Acute care facility (1)

of-life venue that I was not able to observe first hand, it is not clear to me in what specific ways Dutch hospitals are similar to and divergent from American hospitals. Interviews with study participants suggest that compared to the kind of care that is available in the Dutch home, hospital care is more compartmentalized by medical specialty, and less personal, flexible and individualized than home care. Some research suggests that ideal death is thwarted because in certain venues (particularly hospitals), dying individuals are not allowed room for processing meaning (Kaufman 2005; Puchalski 2006) or emotion (Mamo 1999). American physician, Christina Puchalski, finds in American healthcare there is not enough chance to talk about dying. She writes, "[i]n many cases, treatment choices would be different if patients were given the chance to talk about their desires with their physicians long before the deathbed scene. Dying people are not always listened to—their wishes, their dreams, and their fears go unheeded" (Puchalski 2006:5). Medical anthropologist, Sharon Kaufman (2002; 2005), finds something similar. She writes,

> A "time for dying"—with all that idea implies for responding to the humane, facilitating closure of a life,

and allowing a space for finitude and the transcendent—
is difficult to create for the majority of persons who actually are near death, especially within the existing culture and structure of the American acute care facility
(Kaufman 2002:35).

In the Dutch home and in the context of euthanasia discussions
dying individuals are encouraged by *huisartsen* to process what it
means to die in the company of their family and their *huisarts*.
Emotions are a large part of the experience of dying and in euthanasia talk, fear and uncertainty—two emotions frequently expressed by those who are dying—can be socially processed and
culturally addressed.

   Surrounded by Family. Matthijs' ideal was to die at home staring into his garden, surrounded by family and receiving the kind
of care that his mother would give, that kind of unconditional love
that never has to be paid back. He and David had that kind of unconditional caring relationship. While they did fight at times, the
core of their relationship was based on caring for each other. David
nursed Matthijs through rough times and Matthijs had dinner waiting for David when he came home. One of the most important
life lessons that I learned after time spent with so many who were
dying was that at the end what mattered to most people was their
closest relationships. Who they loved and the relationships they
wish they could repair if only they had acted differently was what
mattered most.

   The Dutch ideal is to die surrounded by family and this was
probably most evident in the stories of what happened when death
was not ideal. One female *huisarts* described to me the difficult case
of a woman with terminal breast cancer who had requested assisted
suicide. Her husband and her son were in support of her request.
Her condition and suffering warranted assistance, but the woman
had had a fight with her daughter 15 years before and even though
they lived only a few houses away from each other, they had not
spoken since. Dr. van den Berg was reluctant to go through with
the request because of this lingering family conflict and, like other

huisartsen I met, attempted to initiate a reconciliation before proceeding with the euthanasia request. The woman's daughter was not willing to reconcile with her mother, and so three weeks after her request the woman died by assisted suicide surrounded by all of her family, except her daughter.

Suffering. The fact is that the kind of conditions that occurs at the end of life, particularly now that people are living longer with more chronic conditions (Lynn 2004), can produce a great deal of suffering. The fallacy is that for every pain, discomfort or suffering there is a pill or a fix, but this is simply not true. And I saw this both in the U.S. and in The Netherlands. I've seen the effects of Huntington's, where a young woman covered in bruises could no longer control any part of her body. She lived in restraints to keep from injuring herself, couldn't speak or effectively communicate, her body bound yet her mind intact leaving her ultimately at the mercy of her caregivers who couldn't understand if she wanted to eat, what she wanted to eat, if she needed private time or wanted to hear that long story about someone's weekend. I've seen and smelled the effects of diseases and infections that rot limbs and flesh, blackened feet and left holes, bedsores, the size of softballs. And I've seen the kind of suffering at the end of life that there is no cure for—nausea, aches, and fever that no longer respond to treatments—and indignities that can only be endured. For some, nothing short of morphine-induced unconsciousness could end their suffering, yet for many people drug-induced unconsciousness is not desirable.

Matthijs' wish to die in his sleep or staring into his garden is an expression of his desire for a painless, ideal death. For Matthijs, there were plenty of examples of bad death to fear. The AIDS virus attacks the immune system, leaving sufferers open to any number of illnesses, sometimes one after another. While many more people are living with AIDS today, Matthijs' case had advanced to such a degree that his body no longer responded to available treatments. Matthijs' parents both had protracted and painful deaths, his father receiving a dose of morphine that ended his life after getting to the point where he was struggling to breathe. Matthijs did not want to die that way and mentioned it several times in our interviews. Then there was David's former partner who also had a long and painful death, suffering badly due to complications from AIDS. Matthijs made it clear to me that he did not want to put David (or himself) through that.

Euthanasia talk provides dying individuals with both an idealistic and realistic image for death. By talking about it, individuals invoke their ideal scenario; an ideal in which they may be situated in the bed overlooking the garden, surrounded by loved ones (not gasping for air, vomiting, in pain, or incontinent). Concepts of the ideal play such an important role at the end of life because they offer an important cognitive defense against suffering, both real and anticipated. The caring *huisarts* arrives, administers the shots and the person drifts off held by his loved ones. By talking about euthanasia and having their ideal death be a real possibility, dying individuals get to live that ideal in the days they have left. If events begin to turn and their suffering actually becomes something they dread, they know that euthanasia can change that and often it is the knowledge (the idea) of euthanasia that makes what does come bearable.

Control at the End of Life

At the core of euthanasia talk and Dutch notions of what makes death ideal, is a tension between cultural striving for order and the (oftentimes) unpredictability of illness and death. When the body is failing, people experience bodily losses and depending on the dying trajectory created by the illness, those losses can occur unexpectedly or stretched out over a period of time. How does that affect the person who is dying? Anthropologist Gay Becker writes,

> Order begins with the body. That is, our understanding of ourselves and the world begins with our reliance on the orderly functioning of our bodies. This bodily knowledge informs what we do and say in the course of daily life (Becker 1997:12).

Bodily distress disrupts the order of the body; it disrupts a sense of self; and it disrupts the stories that people use to make sense of themselves and the world in which they live.

Matthijs talked about issues of uncertainty and control at several different points in our interviews. It was one of the reasons he initiated his euthanasia request. When I asked Matthijs why he wanted euthanasia, he gave me two answers: (1) for use in the event that the future might be uncontrollable and (2) because if it got really bad, he wanted to spare his partner from having to go through that with him. No one knew what suffering the future might hold for Matthijs. His hope was to die in his sleep or staring out into his garden. The best he knew, however, was that he did not want to die the deaths his parents died. Taking control through euthanasia talks was the middle ground between these two extremes.

During the year I knew Matthijs, he had, with David's help, come to exert quite a bit of control over the direction of the remainder of his life. He had chosen to stop all treatment, with some friction from his family about it. He was able to remain living at home, predominantly with the help of David. He also received financial assistance from the government since leaving employed work, had some assistance provided by hospice, and was on the wait list for *Thuiszorg* (Dutch Homecare).[4] In the face of an uncertain future, Matthijs initiated a euthanasia request with his *huisarts*. If his hopes for an ideal death did not occur and his fears of a difficult death became real, Matthijs had at his disposal the choice of having his life end early. When I asked Matthijs how he came to initiate his request for euthanasia, he said it was not because he was afraid of dying; it was because he was afraid of dying "worried" like his parents died. At the end, both received a shot of morphine that helped

---

4. When I met Matthijs he was able to largely care for himself. He was typically up and around, dressed for the day, able to cook and clean. Because of his recent bout with dementia, however, he had agreed not to leave the house on his own. His need for homecare was mainly in the event of a medical setback that might include being bed bound or another bout with dementia.

end their life. Matthijs thought this was the same as euthanasia, but I disagree. They may have had a death similar to a euthanasia death, but unlike Matthijs what they did not have was the advantage of *talking* about euthanasia, of planning for an ideal and experiencing comfort in knowing that someone would help them in the event that suffering became too much. Euthanasia talk gave Matthijs a framework for taking back some control during the course of his illness prior to death, which his parents did not have.

Becker (1997) suggests that in the U.S. there exists a pervasive ideology towards continuity. Americans strive to maintain continuity in their life stories and they use narratives to mediate disruption and disorder. I would argue that continuity is not just an American motivation, Dutch people strive for continuity as well. Euthanasia talk is a kind of narrative that both Becker (1997) and Seale (1998) describe. It is a way that Dutch people to manage bodily and social disruption at the end of life. Euthanasia talk helps dying Dutch individuals maintain order and re-negotiate a sense of self at a time in life when disruptions are often becoming more frequent and more severe, and when present and future are becoming increasingly tentative. Euthanasia talk bridges present circumstances with a future ideal, giving space for processing meaning and reaffirming continuity in the face of disruption.

Maintaining Connection

For Matthijs and nearly every other participant in my study, family and relationships played a prominent role at the end of life. When someone was dying, important relationships were what they valued most. Families made dying at home possible (by providing the round-the-clock care that *Thuiszorg* could not) and families were integral participants in euthanasia discussions. Disruption to social bonds at the end of life is a natural part of the dying process. Dying individuals deal with a series of social losses, particularly when decline is stretched out over time. For the people in my study, this often meant that they could no longer get out on the bicycle or do their shopping and errands. They became homebound and eventually bed-bound. They stopped being able to cook and share meals, clean the house, work in the garden, and as time went on, more and more of their daily self care (bathing, toileting, etc.) had to be done by others.

What happens both in the U.S. and in The Netherlands is that as someone grows sicker, weaker and closer to death, their social circle decreases typically to family and close friends. What is different about The Netherlands, however, is that the social world of the dying individual is not typically limited to the family. It is a social world that includes frequent home visits by *huisartsen* and daily home visits by *Thuiszorg* nurses and personal care attendants. One of the more frequent complaints I heard while in The Netherlands was of "too many strangers" in the home, referring to all the *Thuiszorg* personal care attendants who would visit. In the U.S., for those lucky enough to be able to die at home, there are few supports for home care, so there are typically few to no visits from health care professionals, with the exception of hospice, which does not come by daily, and home health services for some of those receiving Medicaid or for those who can afford to pay for it. In the U.S., one's social world usually shrinks to family or friends who have committed to taking care of you. Matthijs was not yet in need of daily home care, but he was on the waitlist for it and like other participants was likely to receive it if need arose.

Thuiszorg figured prominently at the end of Dutch life. In my sample, more than half (9 out of 17) who lived at home received *Thuiszorg* services. See Table 5.1. I conducted observation with Amsterdam *Thuiszorg* and recall one woman in particular whose social network and daily care relied on *Thuiszorg*. She was an elderly woman, regal and very charming, who had made her mark as an actress. Unlike most patients I met, she did not have family to take care of her but was still able to stay at home to die. Home-bound and bed-bound without anyone else to care for her, *Thuiszorg* employees came by daily to give her food, medicine, bed baths, and incontinence care. Socially isolated, *Thuiszorg* employees also gave the woman limited social support. She had wonderful stories about famous actors and behind-the-scenes events with which she entertained home-care employees. The woman was lonely though and even with the frequent presence of *Thuiszorg*, it was evident that home care workers could not take the place of family and close friends.

What *Thuiszorg* and other home-based services accomplish, however, is to add another type of social connection that is available in the Dutch home and not in most American homes at the end of life. The fact is that in American homes, many are left to make it on their own with the family they have. In The Netherlands, family care at the end of life is supplemented and in many ways supported. With *Thuiszorg*, nursing assistance is available up to four times daily (including overnight respite). Nursing assistance includes setting out meals, self care (bathing, dressing, toileting), help with medications or wound care, and some basic house cleaning. Once signed in with *Thuiszorg*, patients receive a nurse who is responsible for integrating daily nursing and personal care in consultation with the *huisarts*. This person may visit the home daily or several times a week. *Huisartsen* visit the home weekly, daily and sometimes several times in a given day if necessary. In addition, *Thuiszorg* employees will do dishes and straighten rooms; there is a cleaning service that will come weekly to clean the house; and another that will provide meals.

Maintaining social bonds at the end of life is not, however, solely about the presence of other people. Social bonds are maintained by a person's ability to participate in relationships and by the emotional connection that is shared. In the time I knew Matthijs, he was able to participate in his life and in his relationships. He was able to cook and eat, to get out of bed, to read and host visitors even though at times his energy was low and (due to his earlier brush with dementia), he had promised David that he would not leave the home alone. A month earlier, however, Matthijs was in a very different situation when he was hospitalized and eventually isolated in a private room where doctors expected him to die. I asked what that felt like and Matthijs said that at the time he thought, if he wanted, he could let his life go, but he didn't because his relationships were what mattered when death was close. He said his orientation to the world became an emotional one—emotion over rationality—and what was most important was having someone who cared for him and loved him. Being able to express love and caring even when most social activities are no longer possible keeps people connected and can be one of the remaining characteristics that affirms sociality. Recall the fight over Terri Schiavo in the U.S. From 1998 to 2005, she lay in a persistent vegetative state—awake, eyes open, but without awareness. Her parents saw something more in her eyes, something that affirmed for them her lingering sociality. Sometimes near the end of life a look is all that is left and how that is read by family and healthcare employees can determine the line between social life and social death.

By invoking euthanasia, dying individuals tap into a deeply ingrained Dutch discourse that has grown out of and, when invoked, in turn fosters a Dutch way of life; a collective way of life. When dying individuals enter euthanasia talks, they engage a discourse that heightens and focuses the experience of dying according to a culturally-shared and patterned dialogue that fosters familial and societal relationships. Part of this social network of relationships includes *huisartsen* and homecare in a way we do not see in the U.S. Matthijs and David had had several talks with Dr. de Boers about euthanasia and both were comfortable that they had found the right *huisarts* to help them if the time came. For both David and Matthijs, this belief was important. The relationships that Matthijs and David shared with his specialists and their previous *huisarts* had been difficult. David, as an American outsider and a former nurse, tended to clash with the Dutch system, questioning Matthijs' doctors in ways in which they were not accustomed. By the time I met them, Matthijs had stopped all treatment with his other specialists, David had asked hospice not to return to the house, and Dr. de Boers was the only connection they still maintained with the Dutch healthcare system. While I am not certain that this relationship would stand the test of time, at that point it seemed to be offering what was needed. From David's perspective, euthanasia talk tapped into American narratives of individuality and freedom of choice. According to David, euthanasia talk offered

Matthijs independence and freedom to make up his own mind about how he would die. From Matthijs' perspective, this tapped familiar Dutch narratives. Euthanasia is an end-of-life option to Dutch people. You get a terminal prognosis and you talk about euthanasia. In The Netherlands, euthanasia is a social experience managed by the *huisarts* and engaged in consultation with your *huisarts* and your family.

Euthanasia talk is based on an ideal that favors continuity in personhood and in relationships. Engaging in euthanasia talk gives individuals who are dying an active role that binds them to family and society. Seale states that social death will occur before biological death when one's connections to self and society have been irreparably severed (Seale 1998:7). In The Netherlands, an end-of-life discourse exists to prevent that from happening. Social death need not occur or can be staved off until nearly the end as individuals take active roles in planning their death through euthanasia talk.

Individuals Excluded

It is important to point out that engaging in euthanasia talk does not always empower individuals, or facilitate social bonds or ideal deaths at the end of life. As described in Chapter 2, there are informal and unspoken rules for engaging in euthanasia talk, rules that favor certain people over others, rules that can be broken and those that cannot. From the position of the person making the euthanasia request, there are a number of informal rules that must be followed to successfully engage in euthanasia talk. First, you must have the right kind of illness or disease. Engagement in euthanasia talk favors dying trajectories that have somewhat predictable levels of future suffering and decline. Illnesses must also have some level of predictability in terms of time frame. For example, risk of stroke is not a good reason for a euthanasia request, because it can occur at any time in the unknown future.

Cancer is the most common illness associated with euthanasia requests because of its often predictable decline trajectory and the level of suffering that decline is known to produce. In my case study sample of 14 patients with euthanasia requests, 10 had been diagnosed with cancer. See Figure 5.2. For those without cancer or another illness with a somewhat predictable level of suffering and trajectory of decline, engaging in euthanasia talk becomes more difficult.

Figure 5.2 Main Illness of Patients with
Euthanasia Requests (n=14)

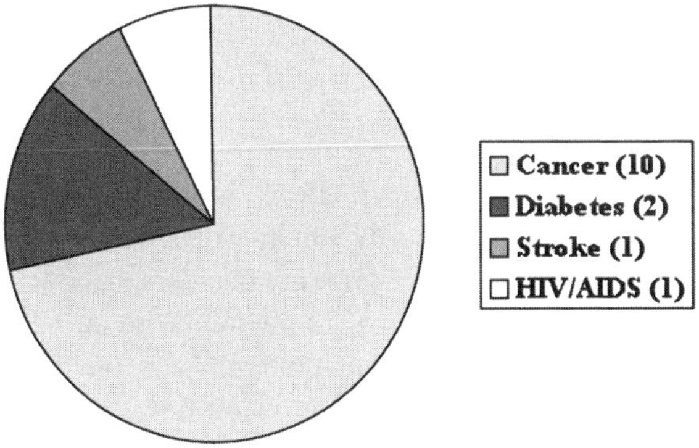

Getting old is not considered sufficient cause for euthanasia. Euthanasia cases tend not to be the oldest of the old, but those suffering from life-threatening illnesses at a slightly younger age. In 2001, for example, 38 percent of those who died by euthanasia were 64 or under, 41 percent were 65–79 and only 21 percent were 80 or older (Wal, et al. 2003:49). In my sample, the mean age for those with requests was 68 compared to 80 for those without euthanasia requests. Of those with euthanasia requests, 7 of 14 persons were in their 50s, with the youngest at age 52. No one with a euthanasia request was over the age of 89. See Figure 5.3.

Finally, engagement in euthanasia talk favors physical illness over mental illness or emotional distress. While one of the more

Figure 5.3 Age Range of Persons with and without
Euthanasia Requests (n=25)

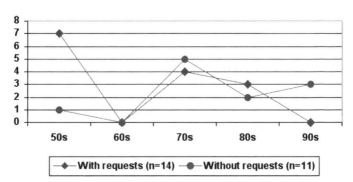

controversial sides to the Dutch law allows for persons with any
kind of illness, not necessarily somatic or terminal, to legally
receive euthanasia, in practice these are the cases that doctors prefer to avoid. In my sample, 2 of 14 persons with euthanasia requests had periodic dementia. One was a woman who had
suffered a stroke and had some confusion but was still deemed
able to decide about euthanasia and the other was Matthijs who
had suffered a bout of dementia due to complications from AIDS.
Both had long standing requests for euthanasia which established a clear-headed request and both were currently either in
remission or not yet terminal. See case studies 7 and 10, Table
5.1.

    In order to maintain euthanasia discussions, savvy individuals
must know what can and cannot be said. Dying individuals who want
to engage in euthanasia talk must not ask to be killed; but they can
be *benauwd* (anxious or short of breath). They should not be severely depressed; they must suffer in appropriate ways (stoically or
with pain medication); and they must remain surrounded by family, not isolated from society. And while David's participation in
this dialogue as a family member is supposed to be an active one,

it was likely that his manner as an American outsider might be cause for future discord if euthanasia discussions progressed. Euthanasia is for Dutch citizens who act in Dutch ways. Matthijs and David's earlier experiences challenging the former *huisarts* and withdrawing from all treatment were behaviors on the borderline of Dutch etiquette.

Not everyone stays connected to social life through euthanasia talk and makes a smooth transition from life to death. Certain people have difficulty engaging in euthanasia talk. Recent immigrants, non-Dutch speakers, Dutch people who break the rules by outrageous behavior or by isolating themselves socially are typically excluded from (or have difficulty engaging in) these discussions. There was, for example, one elderly man from Suriname who went to his *huisarts*, asking in broken English for euthanasia. "Kill me," he said, "I want to die." "Why?" she asked. "For the pain," he said. She continued talking about his pain and sleeplessness when he asked again for her to kill him. That won't be necessary, she replied, writing him a prescription for more sleeping pills. Later she explained to me that he was depressed, not a reason for euthanasia. I suggest that this man, and others I met, did not fit the informal and unspoken requirements for engaging in euthanasia talk.

Being capable of engaging in euthanasia talk also does not guarantee a smooth transition to death. Dying is hard and while euthanasia talk seems to make it somewhat more manageable, more controlled and the burden more shared, it does not take away from the gravity of this time. Matthijs did not want to die. David certainly did not want to lose him. And Dr. de Boer, who had already performed two euthanasia deaths that year, was not thrilled at the prospect of another. But for Matthijs, the thought of going into the uncertainty of the end-of-life without a plan was worse than going into it with this contract between them. However tenuous euthanasia plans are, they are at least something that binds patients, families and *huisartsen* until death occurs either by euthanasia or by other means.

Window to the Garden

Over time I came to see a transition that occurs when Dutch people die at home. It is a transition from watching the neighborhood go by and being watched by neighbors in the front windows of the home to contemplating the garden from a hospital bed positioned at their back window. I return to the theme of Dutch windows and gardens because it strikes me as a metaphor for transitioning from health to disease, from life to death, and from active participants in public space to winding down in Dutch private.

Any new visitor to The Netherlands has noticed the large, curtainless windows of the typical Dutch home in the city and in the country. When I first came to live in The Netherlands, I was surprised that I could walk the streets and have an unobstructed view of people eating dinner, watching the nightly news, or just sitting around their living room. As I entered these Dutch homes in the course of my work, however, I also noted how the front windows were used by those within. It is the pastime of some Dutch people, particularly as they grow older, to sit in their front windows, watching the people and the happenings of the street go by. Swedish anthropologist Ulf Hannerz (and visitor to Amsterdam) suggests that the Dutch window is a device that allows culture to flow from private to public and vice versa (Hannerz 2000:176).[5] Private space does not begin at the door of Dutch homes; it begins in rooms at the back of the house, where neighbors and passersby cannot see you. According to popular legend, leaving windows open to the public is a cultural practice that originated in the 17th century when people left their windows (and their nightly lives) exposed in response to strong Calvinist views that favored proper Dutch behavior. By exposing their nightly routines to the street, who of their neighbors could question their propriety? Legend tells a different

---

5. For more on sociocultural practices of Dutch windows, see Hernan Vera (1989).

story, however, of people disguising alcohol in tea cups for the benefit of their nosy neighbors. Things were not always what they seemed.

Today, when Dutch people get sick a shift often occurs from the front rooms to the back. Before someone grows too weak to get out of bed, they are included in the activities of the living room, watching the street and being watched by the street. When someone who is dying grows weaker, however, *Thuiszorg* comes in and provides them with a hospital bed that is typically situated in a room (usually a dining room or den) on the first floor at the back of the house overlooking (if they have one) the back garden. This is private, intimate space, reserved for family and close friends. This is not a place to be on display to the public. It is a metaphor that comes to rest in Dutch ideals of death — a good Dutch life winding down, coming home to die in the warmth of first floor family life, and in private contemplation of the garden that nature and they together had a hand in making.

Dutch private is not entirely private, however, and the "public" enters even this space in the form of homecare and euthanasia talk. With sometimes daily visits from the *huisarts* and with *Thuiszorg* nurses and nursing aides coming and going the Dutch sick home is far from private. Matthijs was not yet at the stage where he needed *Thuiszorg*, so for him his euthanasia request with Dr. de Boers was the only thing currently keeping him connected with the health care system. Consider, though, what that standing request means. It means that if Matthijs gets sicker and cannot achieve a peaceful death on his own, his *huisarts* will come into his home and take him into death the next best way. This is because Dutch death and the time leading up to it are a matter of both private and public concern in The Netherlands.

Table 5.1 Characteristics of 25 Patients with and without Euthanasia Requests

No. Case	Gender	Age	Marital Status	Main Illness	Prognosis	End-of-Life Location	Home Care Used	Primary Caregiver(s)	Time from Request to Death*	Outcome**
1	Female	72	Married	Cancer	Terminal	Home	No	Husband	10 months	Euthanasia death
2	Female	59	Single	Cancer	Terminal	Home	Yes	Sister/Father	1 month	Natural death
3	Female	82	Widow	Cancer/Aneurysm	Terminal	Home	Yes	Daughter	—	Living
4	Male	80s	Married	Cancer	Terminal	Acute Care	—	Wife/Children	3 months	Euthanasia death
5	Male	74	Married	Cancer	Terminal	Home	Yes	Wife	12 months	Natural death
6	Female	58	Married	Cancer	In remission	Home	—	Husband	—	Living
7	Female	78	Widow	Stroke/some dementia	Not terminal	Nursing Home	—	Son	—	Living
8	Female	57	Married	Cancer	Terminal	Home	Yes	Husband/Children	17 days	Euthanasia death
9	Male	54	Married	Cancer	Terminal	Home	Yes	Wife	17 days	Natural death
10	Male	52	Married	HIV/AIDS/some dementia	In remission	Home	—	Husband	—	Living
11	Female	75	Widow	Diabetes/Kidney failure	Not terminal	Nursing Home	—	Daughter	Unknown	Natural death
12	Male	57	Married	Cancer	Terminal	Home	No	Wife	—	Living
13	Female	55	Married	Cancer	Terminal	Home	No	Husband	5 months	Natural death
14	Male	89	Widower	Diabetes	Not terminal	Nursing Home	—	Children	—	Living

Euthanasia Requests (side label)

Table 5.1 Characteristics of 25 Patients with and without Euthanasia Requests, *continued*

No. Case	Gender	Age	Marital Status	Main Illness	Prognosis	End-of-Life Location	Home Care Used	Primary Caregiver(s)	Time from Request to Death*	Outcome**
15	Female	90	Widow	Non-specific	Not terminal	Nursing Home	—	Daughter	—	Natural death
16	Female	91	Widow	Anemia	Not terminal	Nursing Home	—	Sister	—	Natural death
17	Male	77	Single	Non-specific	Not terminal	Home	Yes	Friend/Sister	—	Natural death
18	Female	91	Single	Cancer	Terminal	Nursing Home	—	None	—	Natural death
19	Female	77	Widow	Cancer	Terminal	Home	Yes	None	—	Natural death
20	Male	52	Married	Cancer	Terminal	Home	Yes	Wife/Brother	—	Natural death
21	Male	87	Married	Emphysema	Terminal	Home	Yes	Wife/Daughter-in-law	—	Natural death
22	Female	79	Unkn.	Cancer	Terminal	Nursing Home	—	Unknown	—	Natural death
23	Male	78	Unkn.	Cancer	Terminal	Home	Unkn.	Daughter-in-law	—	Natural death
24	Female	75	Unkn.	Cancer	Terminal	Home	Unkn.	Son	—	Natural death
25	Male	81	Married	Cancer	Terminal	Home	No	Wife	—	Terminal sedation/death

No Requests for Euthanasia

* The numbers in this column measure the time from the first date of the most recent request phase, often following the patient's terminal prognosis.

** "Natural death" refers to death due to natural causes and "living" refers to patients who were alive at the end of the 15 month study period.

CHAPTER 6

A FAMILY MATTER:
EUTHANASIA IN FAMILIES
AND HOMES

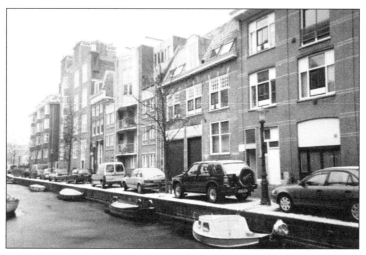

Row of homes in Amsterdam. Photo credit: Frances Norwood

The meaning of home and the relation of home to family has played a central role in cultural practices in The Netherlands and, in particular, in how euthanasia talk occurs at home and with the *huisarts*. Euthanasia talk is not a practice that occurs in social isolation between dying individuals and their *huisartsen*. It is a practice that occurs within families and within the context of home. Euthanasia is a family matter.

The Dutch have created a particular style of "home" that impacts how families have come to relate within Dutch society. The concept of home has a long and unique history in The Netherlands. According to historian Witold Rybczynski (1986), it was in Dutch cities and towns that the home first evolved from the combination live-work space of the Middle Ages to the more intimate, individualized, and family-oriented space that we still see in many European and American homes today. Rybczynski writes,

> [S]ince the Middle Ages, many people no longer lived "over the store," there was a growing number of bourgeois—builders, lawyers, notaries, civil servants—for whom the home was exclusively a residence. The result of this separation was that—as far as the outside world was concerned—the house was becoming a more *private* place. Together with this privatization of the home arose a growing sense of intimacy, of identifying the house exclusively with family life (Rybczynski 1986:39).

The appearance of intimacy in the home was a result of the changing relationships within the family, in particular the relationship of parents to their children. In most families across Europe during the Middle Ages, children were sent away from the home often by the age of seven. Children of the working poor were sent to wage jobs; bourgeois children were sent for apprenticeships; and children from higher classes were often sent to serve as pages in noble homes. By the 16th and 17th centuries, with the growing affluence of the Dutch nation, the number of bourgeois families increased and local schools emerged to replace apprenticeships, resulting in the presence of children at home for a greater part of childhood. Children and home, under the care of the female head of house, became the focal point of Dutch family life.

Rybczynski notes that home was not just a physical space, but also a state of being in the family (Rybczynski 1986:62, footnote). Home helped define family and vice versa. The Dutch have two words for the English equivalent, "family." *Familie* refers to the extended family, which could be any combination of parents, children, grandparents, aunts, uncles, cousins, etc. These are family who may, but more likely do not, share the same household. *Gezin*, on the other hand, refers to one's immediate family, bounded typically by the home space that they share. Children remain in their parent's *gezin* until they grow up, move out and started a *gezin* (and a home) of their own.

Today's *gezin* plays a central role at the end of Dutch life in spite of smaller than average household sizes and the limited composition of many Dutch homes, which typically do not include aging parents (SCP 2001:83). Even though children grow up and leave their *gezin*, The Netherlands is a small country and children often stay in regular contact with their parents. It is not unusual for several generations to live in the same town or to return home frequently for family functions and visits. So while those who are aging prefer to live "independent" of their children, children will often be close enough in proximity to provide on-going support when someone becomes sick or incapacitated at the end of life.

This chapter looks at the consequences of euthanasia talk and the role of family in the context of home and the Dutch state. On the one hand, family has maintained an important (and defining) role in what it means to participate in Dutch life. Families and the home they share continue to shape how people live and die in The Netherlands. While the *gezin* may have shrunk in size and composition, the role that families play at the end of life and the power that they can exert in euthanasia discussions is considerable. On the other hand, the state has had an increasingly powerful role in end-of-life policy, entering the Dutch home to take responsibility for how people die. This chapter is about what it means from the family's perspective to participate in euthanasia talk given these tensions between state and home, public and private.

In the following excerpt, I talk with a man who cared for his wife until her euthanasia death. His is the story of one Dutch family, how they participate in euthanasia discussions and how euthanasia affected their lives.

"Already Gone"

I remember Mr. Veenstra [pronounced VAYN-stra] three months after his wife's euthanasia death, a tall man with white hair and kind, sad eyes. He missed his wife. Mr. Veenstra, in his 70s, is one of those large, but gentle men, who talks softly and walks with a slight stoop to the shoulders, which had the unintended effect of making me feel not so small. I first met Mr. and Mrs. Veenstra in the spring of 2000. After her death that summer, I met with Mr. Veenstra regularly over the course of a year and he told me the story of his life, his marriage, and his wife's death.

They were one of those couples that make you feel good to be around. Through 50 years of marriage, three kids, cancer treatments and remissions, they remained in love with each other. Watching them together and hearing Mr. Veenstra describe their relationship, it was truly as if they were perpetual newlyweds. One day after her death, Mr. Veenstra and I talked about what made their relationship so special.

Frances: I'm glad that I got to meet her.

Mr. Veenstra: Ja, I had a really special woman.

Frances: I think so too. I don't know her so well, but she seemed like a sweet and interesting woman.

Mr. Veenstra: There was once a psychology professor in Amsterdam and he said at the start of his class, there are two kinds of people: cuddlers and those who don't cuddle. Cuddling is for those who find it nice to touch, hold each other and to do things for each other. Some people find it nice to do for each other, others don't. Others prefer to have their own space and to live their own life, more independent. This professor said that if you get married, it is important for cuddlers to marry cuddlers and non-cuddlers to marry non-cuddlers, otherwise it won't work out. Then he asked all the cuddlers to raise their hand. I didn't that day, but I remember the story.

Frances: Let me guess, you were one of the cuddlers?

Mr. Veenstra: Ja, my wife and I were both cuddlers. We loved to be near each other.

Mrs. Veenstra was diagnosed with cancer of the intestines in 1980.
She had a piece of her lower intestine removed and received chemother-
apy treatment, which helped her stay in remission for ten years. In
1990, she was diagnosed with a tumor in her brain, which was suc-
cessfully treated. In December 1998, once again she felt discomfort in
her bowels. She got really sick this time and was in and out of the hos-
pital, but they couldn't find anything wrong with her. Finally, in Sep-
tember 1999, they discovered what was wrong this time—the cancer
was back, this time in her intestines and her liver. After almost 20
years struggling with cancer, she was told there was "niks meer aan te
doen (nothing more to do)." Her doctors thought she had anywhere from
a few weeks to maybe three months to live, so she discontinued treat-
ment and came home from the hospital with the intention to die there.

She didn't die when they expected her to and I got to meet her and
Mr. Veenstra in March 2000 on a house call with their huisarts, *Dr.*
de Vries. On the way over, Dr. de Vries fills me in on her case. He tells
me that Mrs. Veenstra has a written request for euthanasia on file
with him. They discussed it two or three months ago, but she hasn't
mentioned it since then. He thinks she might be changing her mind
about going through with it, so he's not going to bring the subject up
with her today. We knock on the door and Mr. Veenstra lets us in. His
wife is lying in a hospital bed in the living room overlooking the back
garden. As we walk over, she jumps up, energetically trying to get into
a sitting position. She's dressed in t-shirt and pajama pants. We say
hello, shake hands and sit down at a table that is pulled up next to her
bed. The table is covered with magazine clippings of beautiful flow-
ers and colorful things. She is an artist and making collages is her art.

She asks for a shirt to cover up, which her husband goes to get for
her and I notice the skin hanging loosely on her arms and her dis-
tended stomach. You can see the tumor is a large one, underneath the
skin on the right side of her abdomen as Mr. Veenstra helps her slide
her arms into a second shirt. Dr. de Vries asks how she is doing. They
talk about what she's eating and what her specialists at the hospital
have told her. She is eating okay, but seems to have different likes and
dislikes than she used to. Dr. de Vries says that sometimes happens
with cancer. She says her heart has been beating fast. Dr. de Vries

wants to listen to her heart, so Mr. Veenstra helps her take her top shirt off slowly, one arm at a time. Dr. de Vries listens through his stethoscope as she breathes in and out for him. Then he uses the fingers of his hand to push in and around her stomach region. "Does that give you pain?" he asks. It does, particularly on the right side. Dr. de Vries helps her put her shirt back on and sits down again. He thinks it is the cancer, not the medication, making her heart beat fast. He asks if she's up and around at all. "Ja," she says, and she's been outside too. She says her hospital doctor suggested that she do collages because she can't do her other art anymore. "I do it because I like to," she says. They continue chatting, then she gets up to go somewhere. Mr. Veenstra says, "where are you going?" "Oh," she says and sits back down, obviously confused. Dr. de Vries makes an appointment for the following week and we go. In the car he says it is interesting that she didn't mention euthanasia at all this time.

For many months after that, euthanasia did not come up. Mr. Veenstra cared for his wife at home, and as she got sicker he did more and more. They had decided that as long as they were able, they would rather do it without the help of home health nurses. While they did receive supplies (the bed, etc.) from Thuiszorg, *Mr. Veenstra wanted to care for her himself as long as he was able. He cooked for her, bathed her, changed her, and got up with her throughout the night. Near the end, he said, she was taking 28 pills a day and had increasing difficulty with pain, nausea, vomiting and diarrhea. The vomiting and diarrhea became uncontrollable and when she could no longer sit up in bed to do her artwork, they agreed it was time for euthanasia. Ten months after she was told there was* "niks meer aan te doen," *she was ready. I asked Mr. Veenstra when her decision to live became a decision for euthanasia.*

Frances: When did it change?

Mr. Veenstra: Well, that changed slowly. She was so sick, she couldn't paint anymore, then she did collages with clippings. When she couldn't do that anymore, she began writing haikus. See, she was always busy and when she couldn't do that anymore, she wanted to die. Ja, she had written a euthanasia declaration. She'd written that before so we asked Dr. de Vries what we could do about that. Then we had to wait another two weeks, because Dr. de Vries couldn't just do it the next day, he had to prepare.

Frances: And how was that for you? Was it good that he took the time?

Mr. Veenstra: Well, my wife wanted it to be as soon as possible, she wondered why it took so long. But Dr. de Vries had to do it by the regulations and even on the last day, the day of her euthanasia death, she had to sign her declaration for euthanasia again, but she couldn't because she was so weak.

Frances: Did she use morphine?

Mr. Veenstra: Ja, not the patches but the pills and later when she couldn't do the pills anymore, she used suppositories. She didn't want to use the morphine though because it made it hard to think. Then we didn't have good contact with each other anymore and she said she would always prefer pain over being out of her senses. We did use it when it was bad. When she had so much pain and she was so sick, then it was necessary. But that was something we could always discuss and decide together.

Frances: And what did you do with her in this time?

Mr. Veenstra: I just cared for her. She had so much pain, so she slept a lot. I was really busy. She took something to prevent constipation, which gave her constant diarrhea. Her bed was often wet with it, the floor too. So I was always doing the washing, cleaning the floor and the toilet. She was ashamed of that—that was so sad, because she no longer had control. She often vomited.

Frances: I remember in March when I talked to you both, I asked her why euthanasia and she said that she had her art and as long as she could do her art, that's what she would do.

Mr. Veenstra: Ja.

Frances: When did that change?

Mr. Veenstra: Ja, we were both ready. We were ready two weeks before. I could always talk really well with my wife. We had a good marriage. We loved each other very much and the children too. We have wonderful children and good contact among us. But the last two weeks, I had the idea that something in her was gone. My contact with her was lost. Not just because of the morphine, it was the same *when she took no morphine. It was like a small part of her was already dead.*

Frances: I understand.

Mr. Veenstra: It's like she withdrew and I no longer had that spiritual connection with her. That went slowly away.

Frances: So you mean a piece of her was already gone?

Mr. Veenstra: Ja. And in regards to euthanasia, that is very important. I think euthanasia is a good solution. You have everything in your own hands. When my father died, he lived up north and we went every weekend (150 kilometers). But he didn't die. And we would get phone calls to come immediately because it's going to happen and we came and he kept on living. Six or seven times we came back because we thought, "now this is it," but then nothing happened. With euthanasia you have that in hand. It's organized. The kids were there, because I know how terrible it is to keep coming back, to wait and nothing happens. In the end, my father died without us there. My father was very sick, and he too wanted to die, but in his time euthanasia was not possible.

Frances: Do you think euthanasia is a natural death?

Mr. Veenstra: No, it's no natural death, but it is a good death. It is ultimately the end of your life. If you can organize that with others, it is better than if you let it run out. That way you don't know how it might go. I could care for my wife up until the last moment, but if I didn't know how much longer it would be then maybe I would need help. That is important too.

Frances: You mean that the best scenario is to be able to plan?

Mr. Veenstra: Ja, we wanted to take care of it ourselves. We wanted to be able to regulate it ourselves, to be able to say we want it this way and that, because this is obviously an important moment. We were lucky that we could always organize our own lives, like we wanted.

In the weeks and months following his wife's death, Mr. Veenstra had to find new ways to relate to his friends and his world now that he was a widower and no longer a couple. The house became quiet. Slowly the hospital bed and the left-over equipment disappeared. The kids visited regularly and his days were marked by errands out on the bicycle, reading books, and sending e-mails. One of my last visits with Mr.

Veenstra, he surprised me with a story about his wife's ashes. We had been talking about her funeral and how they had organized it to be reflective of her personality, then Mr. Veenstra jumped in with this story.

Mr. Veenstra: I went with the kids to distribute her ashes not long ago. When she was alive, we found a little piece of land in the country where we planned to throw our ashes. This place is really beautiful, with gentle hills and trees everywhere.

Frances: So you were going to distribute her ashes there?

Mr. Veenstra: That's what we wanted, ja. My wife and I picked the place together. But when I went to go pick up the ashes, the funeral company had them a long time, so when I could finally pick them up, I was so happy, that I couldn't get rid of them. So I'm keeping them here, in the house.

Frances: And you didn't throw some of them in the place you picked?

Mr. Veenstra: No, because it is sealed, so I can't get them out. If you open the seal then I'll have to empty the whole thing. I talked to the kids and told them I wanted to keep them safe with me. And when I go, then we can be distributed together.

Frances: So if you die then your kids will distribute your ashes together.

Mr. Veenstra: Ja, and having the ashes here has been a relief. I feel like she's with me now, because before I would come home and the house was empty. Now it's not.

Frances: She's here?

Mr. Veenstra: Ja, [he said pointing to a jar on the bookshelf].

Frances: [Looking around] I think with her art she is also here, but the ashes maybe that is something else.

Mr. Veenstra: Ja, maybe the art is the spirit and the ashes are the body.

In this excerpt you may see many of the themes that were raised in earlier chapters revisited: concepts of ideal death, control, and social death. This story, however, adds another dimension to understanding end-of-life care in The Netherlands, namely the role of the family. Mr. Veenstra's is such a beautiful story about a man who loved and cared for his wife a great deal. Although their story is their own, in many ways Mr. Veenstra's story touches on themes shared by others in my study as well. Family and close relationships are important to people at the end of life. Family members were prominent in nearly all euthanasia discussions that I encountered and family support was instrumental in allowing someone to die at home. Clearly, family and home play an important role at the end of Dutch life. Mr. Veenstra's story demonstrates some of the many ways that the Dutch government enters family life, by euthanasia policy, state welfare, and home health programs. This story also demonstrates some of the ways that euthanasia talk is used within the family and, in particular, how euthanasia talk is used within the family to manage memories and relationships at the end of life.

In the following sections, I will consider (1) how euthanasia talk and end-of-life care is embedded in the context of family and home; (2) how family and the state seem to work largely in cooperation with each other within the context of euthanasia talk and end-of-life care; and (3) how euthanasia talk is used by families to manage memories and relationships at the end of life. I will explore when euthanasia talk by family members does not facilitate ideal death. Finally, I will examine the context of home and how euthanasia talk may be impacted by the venue in which this end-of-life discourse occurs.

A Family Matter

Like most participants in this study, family members played a key role in caring for persons who were dying as well as participating in their end-of-life discussions. Mr. Veenstra made it possible for Mrs. Veenstra to die at home, caring for her around the clock particularly in the last few months of her life. I conducted participant observation with *Thuiszorg* and found that while their services are extensive, even they cannot care for people in the home who are seriously ill without at least some support from another caregiver and typically this means family members. Mrs. Veenstra, like 12 of 14 dying individuals who participated in my study,[1] was able to die at home because she had at least one family member to aid in her care. The more complex the illness and treatments, the more important family become in caring for loved ones at the end of life. See Table 5.1, Chapter 5.

From Mr. Veenstra's perspective, his wife's end of life choices for pain management, euthanasia, etc. was a family matter. They had been a couple for 50 years and it was as a couple that they considered when and how much morphine to use, where their ashes would be spread when they died, and if euthanasia was right for them and for her. Recall what Mr. Veenstra said about how they worked as a couple to manage her use of morphine. She did not want to take morphine because it made it "hard to think." When that happened they did not have good contact with each other, something that both of them valued. He said she preferred pain over the dulling effects of morphine and that that was something that they (and many other families in my study) discussed and decided together.

Under Dutch law, it is up to the dying person to make the decision for euthanasia, but in the discussions prior to death it is a choice that is made in consultation with and consideration of family members as well as physicians who always have the final say of whether or not a euthanasia request meets the requirements for a legal euthanasia or assisted suicide death. Mrs. Veenstra initiated a request for euthanasia after talking to her husband and her family about it. While her *huisarts* and every other *huisarts* with whom I worked urged patients to talk about their request with family, even without urging Mrs. Veenstra and others would have consulted the people most important to her. She consulted them for all of her other

---

1. Of 17 patients who were terminal or actively dying, 14 were able to stay at home to die and 12 of these had at least one family member giving daily care. Only one patient was able to stay at home with only the support of home care services. One patient's family situation was not known. See Table 5.1, Chapter 5.

major healthcare decisions, so it is not surprising that she would include them in one of the most critical decisions at the end of life.

Medical anthropologists and sociologists have paid considerable
attention to conflict that arises between family and the medical establishment as patients and families negotiate end-of-life choices
(Anspach 1993; Glaser and Strauss 1968; Kaufman 1998), but less
attention on the instrumental role of family in end-of-life care. Like
other healthcare choices, the choice for euthanasia in The Netherlands is not made in social isolation. Social bonds are what hold
people to life and in euthanasia talk social bonds are what continue
to hold people to the life they have remaining. Ultimately Mrs.
Veenstra chose to die a euthanasia death, but that was after 20 years
of living with cancer and 10 months after she was told she was not
going to live much longer. Mrs. Veenstra lived well beyond expectation. It is not possible to say what makes some people live longer
than others despite the odds, but it is clear that Mr. and Mrs. Veenstra chose a course of palliative care that maximized what they
found most important (her ability to create art and their ability to
connect with each other) at the expense of minimal management
of pain and nausea. She lived as an active member of her family
and it was only in the last two weeks when she could no longer
maintain her body or her relationships, when "a small part of her
was already dead" that she and her family chose euthanasia.

Family and the State

In the U.S., doctor-patient-family relationships are marked by conflict and individuals and families at the end of life receive few supports to allow them to die at home. In The Netherlands, conflicts
exist, but not in the same way. Conflict in The Netherlands occurs
less often and typically centers on a personality conflict. In the U.S.,
conflict is systemic to medical practice and the doctor-patient-family relationship. American distrust of authority extends quite clearly
to the medical establishment, demonstrated by the patient's rights

movement which pits the concerns of patient and family against concerns of physicians and the healthcare system.

Much of the reason that family can play such an important role as caregivers at the end-of-life is because of the health and social safety nets that exist in the Dutch system. Remember that Mrs. Veenstra had been treated for cancer off and on for over 20 years. She had been sick for much of her adult life and each time she fell ill, Mr. Veenstra cared for her, supported in part by the vast system of social welfare that is available in The Netherlands. Dutch people have numerous supports that can be used when someone in the family is ill. In 2001, nearly 100 percent of the Dutch population had health insurance, approximately two-thirds covered by *Ziekenfonds* (the Dutch health insurance fund) available on a sliding scale fee to anyone who made below a certain wage, free-of-charge for those who could not afford to pay, and with the rest covered by private means. In 2006 in The Netherlands, approximately 72.2 percent of the cost of health care was covered by social health insurance, 8 percent was paid for by patients, 6.8 percent by private insurance, and an additional 13 percent by government and other unspecified sources (CBS 2007:99–100).

In addition to health insurance there are a number of social safety nets included in the Dutch system. In 2006, social health insurance covered approximately 66.8 percent of welfare costs (including extraordinary medical costs for persons who are elderly or disabled), 11.8 were paid for by patients, and 21.4 were covered by government and other unspecified sources (CBS 2007:99–100). The Sickness Benefit pays 100 percent of an employee's wages for the first six weeks of illness and up to 70 percent for the remaining 52 weeks. According to the Disablement Benefits Act (WAO), after the first year if someone is still not able to return to work sick employees can receive up to 70 percent of their former income. The Dutch unemployment benefit system covers those who are eligible at 70 percent of former wages for up to six months and there are provisions for employed workers to take what is called "care leave" to care for sick family members (de Vries 1998:206–210; Griffiths, et al. 2008:15–23; Palriwala 2001).

Health and social safety nets create a secure environment for end-of-life care in The Netherlands, providing dying individuals and their families with a number of key supports. The Dutch system is not, however, without its weaknesses. Some would argue that the system has its faults and the family-state relationship cannot wholly be characterized as a cooperative. Waitlists, for example, are the norm, although persons who are terminally ill who demonstrate need are typically moved up on waitlists and everyone in my study who needed home-based services was able to receive them. There are also those that do not agree with how the system functions. In a recent study, Dutch psychiatrist Boudewijn Chabot estimated that between 1999 and 2003, an average of 3.2 percent of all deaths each year could be attributed to "auto-euthanasia," death by stopping eating and drinking (2.1 percent) or by use of sleeping pills (1.1 percent) (Chabot 2007:106). Chabot examined 144 cases of auto-euthanasia for specific characteristics. He found that almost half of all cases occurred after denial of a request for euthanasia by a physician (49 percent), a number of cases that indicated psychiatric illness (10 percent)[2] or no serious illness at all (26 percent), and a large number of cases where it was predicted the patient would have lived one month or more (79 percent) (Chabot 2007:121, 131, 133). Chabot's study includes a sample of people who fall outside of the mainstream, persons who push on towards assisted death by a lethal dose of medication without the full support of family or the Dutch medical system. Compared to my sample, these represent cases of persons who, for various reasons, were not able to or not interested in getting euthanasia by legitimate reasons. These are the types of cases that demonstrate what occurs when someone is not able or willing to follow more mainstream end-of-life discourses and these are the cases that demonstrate when

---

2. The percentage of psychiatric illness cases can be calculated by adding the number of psychiatric diagnoses with stopping with eating and drinking cases (n=5) with overdose by sleeping pills (n=10) divided by the total number of auto-euthanasia cases (n=144).

family and state are no longer in cooperation, something which according to Chabot's study occurs in 3.2 percent of all deaths each year in The Netherlands.

In some ways, it has been suggested that the Dutch state has usurped family roles, including those roles at the end of life. Indian anthropologist Rajni Palriwala and colleagues (2000; 2001) conducted research in The Netherlands regarding the impact of the Dutch social welfare system on relations within marriage, family and other social networks. Palriwala et al. (2000) argues that the Dutch social welfare state grew over the last 50 years to the extent that the state came to bypass certain family roles and responsibilities. By providing so many material supports, the state has inadvertently impacted the emotional content of family relationships and the connection that family members share. In response to this criticism, the state is now placing increased attention within the public sphere on strengthening "social connectedness" and reviving "family values" (Palriwala 2000).

Compared to the U.S., however, the Dutch relationship of family-to-state is quite simply more cooperative and euthanasia talk has emerged in such a way that families and the home space is central to these end-of-life discussions. Even though there is no mention of the role of family in the *Termination of Life on Request and Assisted Suicide (Review Procedures) Act* (2002), family have at the urging of the *huisarts* come to play an instrumental role in euthanasia talk. Mrs. Veenstra needed the input and support of her husband and her children as she contemplated euthanasia. Dr. de Vries also needed her family's input and support to maintain discussions and for his own piece of mind that no red flags such as depression or family conflict existed that would cause him to want to stall or refuse the request. Dr. de Vries needed family participation in order to establish consensus around Mrs. Veenstra's decision for euthanasia, because when family members object to euthanasia it is often taken as an indication by *huisartsen* that all may not be right with the request.

Consensus building through the common Dutch practice of *overleg* (consultation) is what Dutch people do when faced with a de-

Figure 6.1 Reasons for Canceling a Euthanasia Request (n=11)

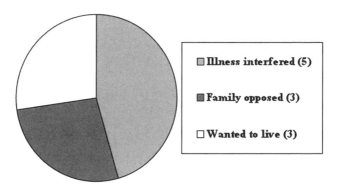

☐ Illness interfered (5)

■ Family opposed (3)

☐ Wanted to live (3)

cision. In Mrs. Veenstra's case, no one in her family objected to her choice for euthanasia. However, in 3 of 11 cases of persons with euthanasia requests in my study sample, a euthanasia request was cancelled due to objections by family members, which was one of three main reasons why a euthanasia request did not end in euthanasia death. The other two reasons were when an illness either progressed too quickly (or went into remission) or when a dying person simply chose to remain living as long as possible. See Figure 6.1.

Managing Memories and Maintaining the Family

Euthanasia talk facilitates ideal Dutch deaths and is used as a means to manage both memories and relationships at a time when relationships and personhood are slipping. Recall Mr. Veenstra's story. I asked him when the decision had been made to go through with euthanasia and he said it was when his wife could no longer create art. At first, she made big, beautiful tapestries. When she became very ill, she switched to making collages from pictures she clipped from magazines. Finally, when she could no longer sit up, she wrote haikus. He also said that in the last two weeks when she could no longer create and had uncontrollable pain, vomiting and diarrhea "it was like a small part of her was already dead." I had heard these words before, both from the man in my opening chapter who felt a photo was a better representation of his dying wife and from the woman whose husband had fallen into a coma after a severe bicycle accident. After the fall, she said he was not the same. "My husband wasn't there. My husband, he's there in the photo," she said pointing the picture. What Mr. Veenstra's and these stories speak to is how identities change when people are dying and how family members who are left behind perceive these changes. When does a photograph become more real than a person? It happens when a person can no longer participate in a relationship and when the memory of that person from the photograph overtakes the personhood of the body in the bed. There is simply something about a person's spirit or essence that sometimes dies before their bodies do. This is social death and this is what invoking an ideal through euthanasia talk and in some cases euthanasia death at the end of life attempts to address (Seale 1998:7–8).

Just as social death can occur prior to biological death, life can linger in the aftermath of death as well. End-of-life rituals have long been associated in anthropology with the management of life after death (Douglas 1966; Gennep 1908; Stewart and Strathern 2003; Turner 1967). Managing memories and relationships with the dead is the work of survivors. Recall Mr Veenstra's comments about his wife's ashes. When he brought her ashes home, he said it was like the house was no longer empty. This is because Mr. Veenstra was able to re-assign personhood (the memory of her person) in part to the ashes left behind. He chose to hold on to her ashes after her death, naming her art as the embodiment of her spiritual body and her ashes as the embodiment of her physical body.

Regardless of whether a euthanasia death occurs, the ideal invoked through euthanasia talk, helps structure the memories that are left for survivors. *Huisartsen* see their role at the end of life to be there for the patient, but also to help manage memories for surviving family members. Dr. Rohmer from Chapter 4 said,

> *Ja*, for me euthanasia is really about communication, not only with folks who are dying but also with those who are intimately involved with the dying person and that is happening more and more. When I first did it that was not the most important aspect but that has grown to be more important. When I am busy with it I think more and more about the bystanders, about the people who remain behind and what it means for them.

Within euthanasia talk there is room for family members to negotiate shifting identities, personhood and relationships as they watch their loved one experience bodily decline and social losses. Consider all that Mrs. Veenstra suffered. Years struggling against cancer, then the final 10 months which ultimately ended in pain, vomiting, diarrhea and disconnect and then an additional two week wait for euthanasia. Yet compared to Mr. Veenstra's father's death, his wife's death was still beautiful.

At several points in my interviews with Mr. Veenstra he kept returning to his father's death. Something about that haunted him. We were talking about how his wife withdrew near the end and how he "no longer had that spiritual connection with her." Mr. Veenstra suggested that euthanasia was a "good solution" for that. Why? [Because] "you have everything in your own hands" and he proceeded to tell me about what didn't go right in his father's death. His father's death was not well scripted because his death was long, painful and drawn-out; it was unpredictable and ultimately occurred without family present. While Mrs. Veenstra certainly suffered near the end, her suffering was made bearable somehow in Mr. Veenstra's mind because together they already had a story with an acceptable ending, whether or not they chose euthanasia at the end. Together they could maintain their family connection and exert some control over their last months and days together, something his father could not. Both suffered and both died with some assistance, but in his father's case, there was no guarantee of assistance prior to death. Something in that guarantee and in that process of formulating the present around an ideal future makes the one death beautiful and the other not.

When Euthanasia Talk Does Not Bring Ideal Death

It is important not to think of euthanasia talk as something that always works to facilitate social bonds or ideal deaths. Engagement in euthanasia talk is a discursive practice that is constantly changing. It is in continual negotiation by those who invoke euthanasia talk as a discourse and among other competing end-of-life discourses, which in The Netherlands include Calvinist stoicism or local dialogues about what *sterke* (strong) men and women do. Much of Dutch life is based on a collective ideal with *gezin* (family) central, yet nuclear families are changing and social isolation does clearly occur in The Netherlands. With more people living longer, the shrinking of extended family networks into the smaller *gezin,* and with more people dying in an institution than at home, isolation is going to remain a clear threat as Dutch people age. Han van der Horst finds a growing trend of isolation among the elderly in The Netherlands (Horst 2001:228–231).

My research supports that. I recall a number of persons, particularly those living in nursing homes, telling me how difficult it was to watch their closest friends and family die. One of my favorite interviews was with Mrs. Bloem. At 91 years old, she lived in a nursing home after watching many of her family and friends die. Her husband died of heart disease at age 77 and over the course of her lifetime she had lost her parents and three of four siblings. Her one remaining sister fortunately lived in the same nursing home. They visited one another daily and received periodic visits and flowers every Friday from an extended family member. She was happy, but isolated—no question her social circle had shrunk. While Mrs. Bloem and her husband had been very social and had known many of their neighbors, she kept mostly to herself at the nursing home. With all the water she drinks, she says she has to go to the bathroom a lot making joining the knitting club and other activities there difficult.

Isolation also occurs when individuals isolate themselves from family or are in conflict with family. In the course of my study, I met a number of people who were estranged or had conflict with family members. Several times I was told of *huisartsen* who initiated calls to estranged family members attempting to facilitate a reunion prior to death and each time there was an estranged family member in the case of a euthanasia request that request was always stalled to at least discuss the possibilities of reconciliation.

The Netherlands has up until the last few decades been a fairly homogenous society, but with the influx of new immigrants from Africa and Europe and refugees from former colonies of Suriname, Indonesia and the Dutch Antilles, The Netherlands is transforming. The transformation, however, has not been as smooth as the Dutch stereotype of "tolerance" and the long standing tradition of being open to foreign trade would suggest (Horst 2001:271–311). In my study, I saw foreigners who were not familiar with Dutch norms and manners isolated, especially when they could not speak Dutch well. Mr. and Mrs. Veenstra were in many ways a typical Dutch family. Matthijs and David from Chapter 5, however, were not. Compare their experiences and you will see some striking differences. Recall Matthijs and David—Matthijs, a gay Dutch man married to David, a man from the United States. While Matthijs and David were gay, not a common conception of "family" in The Netherlands, I believe that Matthijs' marriage to a foreigner probably had the greatest impact on how they were perceived as a family. Traditional Dutch families either assimilate foreigners or they are not considered to be a traditional family. David's American orientation to the Dutch system often left the couple in conflict over Matthijs' care. They had largely isolated themselves from Matthijs' family and had also chosen to isolate themselves in part from the Dutch healthcare system (by refusing all medical treatment with the exception of Matthijs' standing request for euthanasia). In a society that revolves around consensus building, it is okay to be different and to express yourself. It is not okay, however, to fail to participate in the process of building consensus and it is not okay to fail to conform to Dutch ways of acceptable behavior and expression (Horst 2001:181, 249–250). Because in large part David did not conform to Dutch standards of what constitutes family in The Netherlands and because the Dutch healthcare system did not conform to David's standards of proper healthcare, he and Matthijs had experienced a series of conflicts with Matthijs' doctors and were likely to continue to experience some conflict as their euthanasia talks progressed.

When people are connected to family, euthanasia discussions still may not be without conflict. When family members object — and object strongly — euthanasia requests typically do not go through. I met Mrs. Van Dam early on in my study and got to know her over the course of many visits. She was 82 years old with cancer of the esophagus. She had gotten so far as to schedule a date for euthanasia and then canceled it on the day she was to die. I asked her and her *huisarts* separately why she cancelled her date with euthanasia and both of them agreed that it was because she had been pressured by her daughter to call it off. Her daughter was not yet ready to lose her mother. Before her cancellation, Mrs. Van Dam said she wanted euthanasia because her suffering was "unbearable,[3]" her life was no longer meaningful, and she did not want to be a burden to her daughter. Six months later, I asked Mrs. Van Dam what she thought of her decision to cancel her request. She told me during the night she regretted that she did not go through with euthanasia, but when her granddaughter visited she felt differently. She said she was okay with her decision.

This chapter has been about the presence of family at the end of life and in euthanasia discussions. Family is central to Dutch life

---

3. "*Ondraaglijk* (unbearable)" is the term used in the Requirements for Due Care in the *Termination of Life on Request and Assisted Suicide (Review Procedures) Act* (2002). It is also the term you will hear used by physicians and dying individuals attempting to establish the legal requirement that the patient's suffering is "lasting and unbearable."

and to discussions about Dutch death. Their presence (and their absence) makes a difference. When family members do not participate or when individuals become isolated from family, *huisartsen* are more reluctant to enter euthanasia discussions. When family members do participate, they have more power to sway the decisions of their loved one and the opinion of the *huisarts* than is currently understood. Their absence in euthanasia law does not translate to an absence in euthanasia practice. Their ability to participate in *overleg* (consultation) of a euthanasia request allows Dutch *huisartsen* to spread the difficult and highly subjective task of determining "unbearable and lasting suffering" among several integral participants. This is not to say that *huisartsen* do not take responsibility for ultimately determining whether or not to go through with a euthanasia death, but it does mean that they take some comfort in the *process* that has emerged to manage end-of-life decision-making.

Euthanasia in the Context of Home and Family

Earlier in this chapter, I talked about the mostly cooperative relationship between the Dutch family and the state as it relates to end-of-life care. I think a better way to understand exactly how this differs in The Netherlands is to focus on the context of the home versus the institution. The venue in which these healthcare discussions and healthcare relationships occur is important. In a U.S. study of home care, anthropologist Andrea Sankar finds that

> the context exerts a tremendous influence on what transpires between physicians and patients: it can strongly 'dictate' power relationships, what kinds of information are visible or invisible, and how physicians and patients know and experience each other (Sankar 1988:155).

Betty Hasselkus (1994) also looks at the role of context in her study of U.S. family-provider relationships as patients transfer from hospital to home. She finds that as patients move from hospital to home, the power dynamic shifts between providers and family. In the hospital, it is the health provider whose expertise is dominant, the one who knows the patient (or better, the patient's illness) best. In a successful transfer of the patient to home, however, family members now educated by the healthcare professional on the illness and educated on the how-to's of day-to-day care by their own hands-on experience in the hospital come to hold the role of care giving experts at home.

In The Netherlands, more than one-quarter of those who died in 2003 died in their own home (CBS 2004). In The Netherlands, home has retained a power and a place at the end of Dutch life that is less evident in the U.S. Home in The Netherlands is still integrally connected to family and families (*gezin*) have retained a considerable role at the end of Dutch life. Home is where public and private meet in The Netherlands. As I suggested in my last chapter, not only does the public enter through the curtainless windows from the street, but it enters the home via Dutch homecare (*Thuiszorg*) and home visits by the *huisarts*. Dutch people typically do not die alone. Instead they are surrounded by family and home services, and if necessary, by a type of institutional nursing care that emphasizes participation in coffee hours, clubs and other social activities. Through public assistance, home care, and general practice the Dutch state has maintained Dutch citizens through life and now, with the option of euthanasia death and euthanasia talk, the Dutch state also plays a role in maintaining citizens up through and into death. The Dutch state enters the home via euthanasia talk, but has done it in a way that largely fosters family involvement and family relationships.

PART III

CONCLUSION

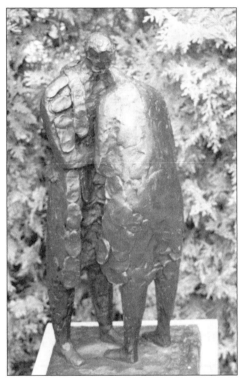

Photo credit: Frances Norwood

The Phone Rings

The phone rang for me in May 2001 and days later I left Amsterdam for a hospital in Florida. My mom had cancer of the colon, large intestine and liver. Like Mr. Veenstra, I, too, am a cuddler so the first thing I did was crawl in bed with her, hugging her small and unsteady frame. She seemed so shaky and frail, and I think I felt like my hugs could keep her grounded, give her life even when we both knew she was dying. My parents did not have health insurance. My father had had two mild heart attacks in his late 30s, so for much of our lives he struggled to keep us insured, paying higher premiums for what was quickly labeled his "pre-existing condition." Finally after the children grew up and left home, he could no longer afford the payments and both my parents made the decision to cancel their health insurance. They decided then that should one of them become seriously ill, they would not seek care. We grew up in a family who rarely went to doctors. Mom was the family's physician, using herbs and home remedies to treat the majority of our childhood illnesses. So when she fell ill, it took a long time before she went to see a physician about her symptoms. By the time she did, it was too late. They opened her up and found tumors that had metastasized to such an extent that treatment would only prolong the inevitable. They took some of her cancer and left her with a ragged scar spanning across the length of her belly held together by staples.

Two days after I arrived in Florida, my mother, the matriarch of our family at 4 foot 11 and only 63 years old, came home to die and I came home to care for her. My dad who at his age should have been nearing retirement needed to keep working during the day to keep the household going. I called hospice and the nurse came over to set us up with the drugs we would need. After experiencing Thuiszorg, *it was shocking how little help is available to Americans who want to die at home and how prevalent the issue of money is in healthcare decisions to those who don't have an extensive system of welfare to back them up. Thank goodness for what hospice could do and luckily for now, dad had his job and mom could still move around on her own.*

As it turned out we had four weeks together before she died. The first week home was rough. She barely ate and was often in pain, but the nausea was worse. The way my mother described it, the pain could be cut back by the morphine to the point where she knew she still had pain but did not mind that it was there. The nausea, however, was different. It never fully went away, no matter what she tried. We had pills, patches and suppositories and our days were marked every two to four hours with the medication regime. We made a chart to keep up with it. Some nights I slept on a mattress at the foot of her bed, other nights she preferred to be alone. She needed her space and she wanted us to have our rest, but I could tell the nights were the hardest for her. The nights were when it was just my mother and the reality of her death alone. On the weekends, family came to visit. My sisters and my brother all took turns visiting. Our mother was dying and we were devastated.

During the week, I had mom mostly to myself. Dad and I gathered around her bed in the morning, and then Dad went off to work for the day. Usually I stayed with her awhile after he left and we talked and enjoyed the view from her bed of the back yard with all the beautiful flowers and plants. She was an artist and, like everything else she touched, the yard was colorful and funky with flowers and plants arranged around interesting home-made wind chimes, Buddhist statues and meditation areas. We talked about a lot of things. She insisted on being in my study, so we taped a series of interviews about how it felt to die, the effects of morphine, and what had become most important to her in her last weeks.

When we weren't taping, we talked about anything. We talked about family, especially how the other family members were coping with the news, and we reminisced about the fun and outrageous things we had done as a family. Other times I just let her be. We were similar in that we liked to socialize, but we needed our private time, too. Sometimes I went for a short run on the beach, and then came home to sit in the next room reading. Mom mostly stayed in her bed and called for me when she needed something.

Not knowing when she would die was difficult. Time seemed to linger between the immediate—dealing with the nausea and the pain, wanting her to eat, keeping up with the medication schedule—and an uncertain future—what would I do when she died, I mean that moment, that day, how would I function without my mother? I couldn't get that far. Since we didn't know how long it would be, I took a job waiting tables on the weekends, something to get me out of the house two nights a week.

After the first week, I think some of the fear she had settled down and we got into a routine. During the week, she went through her old papers and letters, throwing out things that were no longer necessary or too private to leave behind. We also wrote her Last Will and Testament and started planning the party that we would throw for her after she died. Mom wanted something festive and she thought it would be good to have us bring a lot of her artwork so that friends could take something home with them.

Two things really changed for my mom once she knew she was going to die. I asked her what frightened her about dying and she said when she got scared it was not fear for herself, but fear for how her family might feel when she leaves. She didn't want us feeling unresolved about anything, so her four weeks was largely spent trying to give to each of us what she thought we needed most. The other thing that changed for her was her ability to stay in the moment. As a long-time practitioner and teacher of Buddhism, she had always attempted to live in the moment. Now she really was. She explained,

Now I'm seeing things as having an ending. Every morning I wake up, it's another morning that I didn't know if I'd have or not. It's a beautiful morning and the beauty is more alive and real than the beauty I was seeing before because it's not overlaid with concepts of what I ought to do or what it ought to be or what I want it to be or what other people might want it to be. It doesn't have any of that. It just is. So you start seeing it without these little parameters. And when you hear people talk it's so strange because they seem to be talking about a lot of things that don't matter. In the other world I used to live in I would go along with it, but now I don't have to put up with that. I don't want to waste my time with stuff that is junk, that isn't going to get resolved; that isn't going to make people happy. Just let the world happen, watch it a little bit and it will tell you what it wants and what it needs from you. It doesn't need a whole lot, maybe just a little acceptance, maybe, or appreciation and participation.

My mother died before dawn on June 20, 2001. The rest of the family were on their way, but they weren't there. She knew it was coming so the night before she refused all medications. Dying as clear-headed as possible was something that meant a lot to her. In Buddhism, death is an important passage. It is an opportunity to understand the nature of reality and perhaps achieve enlightenment. I knew death was close too, so I sat by her bedside that night to witness the passing of my mother. She was in pain and she was throwing up, so when I could I cleaned around her but mostly I left her alone, which is what she wanted. Next to her bedside, I attempted Tonglen, *a Buddhist practice to take away my mother's suffering while offering her healing light. In her eyes, I could see that she was already on her way. I made a noise and she stared at me for a second or two with hollow, black eyes and in that hollow stare I could see that person that was my mother leaving.*

When the final moments came, I went to get my father. We had agreed that when the time came, my father would be the one to help her die, not by euthanasia or assisted suicide, but by rubbing the crown of her head, where it is thought in Buddhism that the soul leaves the body. We watched her die and then my father did a special prayer to help her on her journey. We cleaned her up and we covered her, and then went in the next room to drink tea and to start making phone calls.

Today, my mother is a memory to me and my family. She is like a good book that I can visit anytime, but the story doesn't change anymore. My father's story, however, is still changing. After my mother's death he did all right. He attempted to date again, to all of the family's dismay. He went on with his life until his stroke. It was massive, but he survived. With the aid of Medicare he spent several weeks in the hospital, and then moved to a rehabilitative unit of a nursing home. Dad didn't have much in savings and still had mom's hospital bills, but after working most of his adult life he had paid off most of his home. Initially, Medicare paid for almost all of his hospital costs— 100 days covered. After that my father paid. Dad required round-the-clock care. He was confused, incontinent, could no longer walk, or do much in the way of self care. When it was clear he would not be physically able to return home and in consultation with my father who

was aware but often confused, we sold his house and the bulk of his
belongings in order to keep him in as nice a place as possible for as
long as possible.

We had researched our options and the options were few. We talked
about bringing him home to one of our houses, but with the amount
of care he needed and the set up at each of our homes it was clear that
that was not going to work. We looked at facilities in Virginia, North
and South Carolina, for something close to one of the four kids. The
nicest places were continuum of care retirement communities, but
these were for people with money who plan ahead. In the continuum
of care facilities we saw, you purchase an apartment connected to an
acute care facility. Then, if you ever get sicker, you have the option of
moving to a higher level of care, as needed. If you didn't buy in initially and in good enough physical condition to largely take care of
yourself, it was next to impossible to get a spot. The wait lists were
enormous for those who had failed to buy one of the apartments and
beds for Medicaid patients were few or not available at all. Most of
the nursing homes that we could afford were awful—white linoleum
floors, and patients parked semi-conscious in the hallways or in front
of their televisions. There was no privacy, something that was important to my father, and the look and feel of these places was institutional. Finally, we found Sunrise Assisted Living, Inc., an assisted
living facility quite different from all the nursing homes we visited,
where dad could live in his own room, decorated with his own things,
and with the freedom to eat and come and go as he liked. A little research revealed that Sunrise was a model of assisted living brought to
the U.S. from The Netherlands in 1981 by Paul and Terry Klaassen.
According to their website,

> [t]he concept of assisted living was familiar to Paul, whose
> grandmothers both lived in comfortable senior homes in
> Holland, where the care and assistance they needed was
> brought to them, delivered in a residential environment.
> As a teenager, Terry and her father struggled to care for her
> terminally ill mother at home [in the U.S.], after they dis-
> covered the only long-term care options were impersonal,

institutional settings. As a result of their experiences and belief that seniors can be cared for and enjoy a quality life, they opened the original Sunrise in Oakton, Virginia (SSL 2003).

Funny that the one place we found ended up being based on a Dutch model of end-of-life care. After having seen so many really frightening nursing homes, Sunrise *was something quite different. I remember the first time I visited the dining hall. There was color on the walls, paintings, carpeting and everyone was seated around small, intimate tables. It looked like a restaurant, not a cafeteria. Residents were given a menu to choose from, with choices of drinks, entrees and deserts. If they didn't want to eat in the dining hall they could eat in their rooms or if they weren't hungry yet, they could always go to the café where food and drinks were available any time of day or night. Imagine having the freedom to eat what you want, when you want. In U.S. end-of-life care, this place was revolutionary.*

We were lucky to find a place that could be a home for dad, but we knew it would be temporary. First, dad was receiving the highest level of care that Sunrise *was able to offer so just one medical setback could send us looking for a new place. Second, our money was going to run out. We had enough for approximately four years of care and after that we would have to find a place that accepted Medicaid. The* Sunrise *where dad lived in South Carolina, like most assisted living, did not take Medicaid patients. We considered the possibility of the four kids pooling our resources together to pay for dad's care when his money ran out, but agreed that that might wipe out our resources as well as my father's.*

In September of 2007, dad had a second but mild stroke, which forced him to leave assisted living. Luckily, we were able to give dad 100 days more of rehabilitation therapy paid for by Medicare, which he enjoyed. Rehabilitation gave him daily visits with physical and speech therapists. It made him feel good to have visitors there just for him and to have a feeling of accomplishment when he made progress in his therapy. This time, however, he had to move out of assisted living to a place that could accommodate his increased need for care.

With his money almost gone, we did not have many options left. We found a place under new management. They had been on the National Nursing Home Watch List for reported incidents of deficiencies with the potential to harm residents and abuses that did harm residents (memberofthefamily.net 2005), but under new management they seemed to be turning that around. They were painting the hallways with some color and many of the nurses and rehabilitation therapists were very kind and personable.

Dad did all right until the 100 days of Medicare funding ended, ending his opportunity to receive daily rehabilitation. His new surroundings were nowhere near as nice as Sunrise and that compounded by the lull in family visits following the holidays sent Dad into a depression. He started refusing meals. For three weeks he refused to eat, growing weaker and eventually ending up in the hospital. My sister Liz who has been closest to Dad and instrumental as a caregiver throughout his institutionalization talked to him. She told me afterwards that he didn't want to die, but he also didn't exactly want to live like this. At Sunrise, he was much more in control of things with his own room and coming and going as he pleased. He doesn't want to be in the hospital and doesn't like experiencing these setbacks, so after his talk with Liz he agreed to start eating again. In February 2008, dad's assets dropped below $2000 and, with the help of an attorney, the first application was submitted for Medicaid. Ten months later he was accepted for Medicaid. He lives today in a nursing home in South Carolina.

CHAPTER 7

Lessons from
The Netherlands:
A Comparison of Practices
and Policies at the End of
Dutch and American Life

The U.S. has a health care system that offers cutting edge treatments for those who have the resources to pay for it. It is a patchwork system that combines the best of palliative care, advanced medical technologies and therapies, with limited but valuable hospice care, outdated models of nursing home care, limited access to home care, and an overall lack of governmental financial supports and safety nets. In the U.S., we favor discourses based on an individual's right to choose, yet clearly those "choices" are limited when you cannot afford to pay. Eventually, everyone must die and what the United States has not been able to do so well is to put together a comprehensive system of care (not necessarily treatment) that encompasses the needs of all Americans at the end of life.

Consider that compared to 30 industrialized nations from around the world, the U.S. is the *only* industrialized nation without universal health coverage (Vladeck 2003). The U.S. has the highest per capita cost of health care in the world, yet 46.6 million people (15.9 percent of the population) remain uninsured (OECD 2006; U.S. Census 2006; WHO 2007). It is shocking to me, particularly after spending time studying Dutch end-of-life care, that we live in a country where my mother would not seek medical assistance until it was too late because of her inability to pay and that my father would end up penniless in a place with not nearly the kind of supports that I know are possible. This is just one story from the U.S., but there are others that indicate that U.S. end-of-life care is in need of fixing (Gleckman 2009; Gass 2004; Daimond 1992; Kaufman 2005; Lynn 2004; Puchalski 2006; Shavelson 1995).

Lessons from The Netherlands

There are lessons we can learn from the Dutch. The Dutch system of end-of-life care, including their euthanasia policies and practices, offers us an important point of contrast to our own system of end-of-life care. What is critical, however, is that before we make such comparisons that we carefully examine the Dutch model for what it means within a Dutch frame of reference. Euthanasia and end-of-life policies and practices cannot be understood, nor transported elsewhere, without understanding what is Dutch about this system. Too many who support and oppose Dutch policies on euthanasia or end-of-life care do so without a clear understanding of how these policies occur in daily practice or are embedded in cultural forms because so few studies are available that detail the day-to-day experience of modern-day euthanasia (cf. Pool 1996; The 1997) or the cultural context in which modern-day euthanasia and other end-of-life practices from The Netherlands occur (cf. Horst 2001; Kennedy 2002). In this final chapter, we will take a broader look at euthanasia and other medical behaviors at the end of life in The Netherlands and the U.S., to consider important lessons this study of Dutch home death can teach us about our own systems of long term and end-of-life care.

Consider Euthanasia Policy in Its Structural Context

One of the first lessons that this study of Dutch policy and practice reveals is the importance of considering any policy in its structural context. Euthanasia and assisted suicide practices are situated in a system of healthcare that is structurally quite different from the U.S. Dutch persons who are nearing the end of life or who are living with chronic illness have an extensive array of services that are available to them, from universal health coverage that includes nearly 100 percent of the population, to coverage for extraordinary medical costs, social safety nets, and a comprehensive system of home healthcare and family supports. Compared to the U.S., the Dutch spend less per capita on healthcare ($2,909 in The Netherlands versus $5,711 in the U.S. in 2003), yet arguably provide much more in the way of services and palliative care (OECD 2006).

In both countries, people spend more time at home near the end-of-life than in the hospital, but in The Netherlands homecare is available to support patients and families, whereas in the U.S. families largely carry this burden alone. When home is no longer a viable option, Dutch people have access to assisted living, nursing homes, 24-hour acute care nursing facilities, and, in a few places, hospice. Compared to the U.S., however, these places tend to have a very different feel. Dutch nursing home rooms and assisted living apartments are typically decorated with the patient's own furniture. Private rooms are more prevalent and the overall feel is more of a home than an institution. Unlike the U.S. nursing homes I entered and left, certain that I would never let any family member stay there, I only encountered one Dutch institution that made me feel that way. It was an independent living group home for people with disabilities, which reminded me of many of the Medicaid-eligible nursing homes I visited in the U.S.

Critics of the Dutch system argue that rationing of healthcare is an inevitable by-product of any universal access system. I agree that rationing does occur in The Netherlands, but it also occurs in the U.S. as well. In The Netherlands, there are waitlists for home-care services, nursing homes, and specialized treatments. Waitlists, however, play a lesser role at the end of life, because when need is clearly indicated patients are moved up on waitlists for services. Not one family in my end-of-life sample failed to receive services requested and this included medical treatments, home care services, respite, and cleaning services. The most common complaint I heard from patients and families in The Netherlands was that there were too many strangers in the home (referring to home health workers). In The Netherlands, the emphasis is on letting the patient choose what is best for them and at the end of life the choices are many. In the U.S., we may not have waitlists per se, but we do have limited health coverage, including limited access to quality housing and homecare, along with complex bureaucratic hurdles that result in sometimes long waits to receive necessary government funding.

Just as in the U.S., families with new diagnoses of terminal illness talk about exploring new, cutting edge treatments but in The Netherlands the shift from treatment to palliative care is more fluid, in part, because in The Netherlands palliative, or comfort care, is already a large part of the existing general practice system for all patients. Compared to the U.S. and Britain, The Netherlands is often criticized for the limited influence of hospice at the end of Dutch life. Critics suggest that without a pervasive system of palliative care, like hospice, euthanasia policy poses more of a threat (Hendin 2002; Zylicz 2002). But it appears that whereas hospice was added to supplement palliative care services in end of life care in the U.S. and elsewhere, these same services already existed within general practice and homecare in the Dutch health care system, where families are given quite a bit of support to die at home and *huisartsen* are much more involved than many of their U.S. counterparts in providing care that extends beyond immediate medical concerns and treatments. Consider that much of Dutch general practice is based in discussion with patients and their family members. Dutch *huisartsen* perform general medical procedures, but also pride themselves on providing medical care for the whole patient. In my sample, I saw *huisartsen* regularly making home visits for the purpose of comforting lonely elderly patients, initiating discussions regarding family relationships and stress in work or marriage, and just playing witness to major life passages, from birth through death.

With the current state of healthcare in the U.S., euthanasia as the Dutch practice it is not a viable option. American general practitioners do not typically practice home-based medicine and do not often have the kind of doctor-patient-family relationship that could currently support a Dutch-style form of euthanasia talk. Americans tend to have a general distrust of authority and a more contentious doctor-patient relationship (Kleinman 1980b; Merelman 1991), which is not conducive to a trust in government to regulate euthanasia policy nor to a trust in physicians to manage such a policy. Offering euthanasia as an option among limited options is risky. Safe euthanasia policy is only viable if it is truly just one option among many.

Evaluate the Enduring Link between Euthanasia and Suicide

In Chapter 3, I looked briefly at the history of euthanasia and its ties with concepts of suicide. Another lesson we can take from this study of Dutch policy is how important it is for any country considering euthanasia or similar end-of-life policies to evaluate, and continue to evaluate, the link euthanasia has shared with suicide. Hitler's programs to euthanize life "not worthy" of life and the resulting Holocaust should continue to serve as a warning to proceed only with caution.

If Foucauldian discourse shapes how people think, feel and act at the end of life, particularly without their full awareness, then it is important to consider whether euthanasia could be an example of a type of failure in the relationship of the individual to society (Durkheim 1951). Could euthanasia talk be compelling complicit

Dutch citizens or citizens without strong ties to Dutch society to die euthanasia deaths? Research suggests generally not. Quantitative evidence from The Netherlands and the U.S. suggests that while people may talk about euthanasia or physician-assisted suicide, only a few are choosing to die legal euthanasia or assisted suicide deaths. Statistics from The Netherlands reveal that each year approximately 1 in 10 who initiate a euthanasia or assisted suicide request with their Dutch physician die an assisted death and between 28 to 41 percent of those who initiated "concrete" requests (requests typically made after serious illness is diagnosed) die by euthanasia or assisted suicide (Onwuteaka-Philipsen, et al. 2007:100, 108; Wal, et al. 2003:46). In Oregon, where physician-assisted dying has only been legal since 1997 (compared to 1984 in The Netherlands), there is quantitative data that suggests something similar. While data is not reported in the same way for Oregon, we find that physician-assisted dying is rare, occurring 341 times between 1997 and 2007 and including less than 1/7 of one percent of all deaths in the year 2003 (DHS 2008). If we look at the number of persons in Oregon who initiate a request for a lethal prescription, we find that between 48 and 67 percent of those who initiate requests die an assisted death, a slightly higher percentage than those who initiate "concrete" requests in The Netherlands (Leman and Hopkins 2004:5). See Tables 2.1 and 3.2.

What these figures do not reveal, however, are cases of *il*legal euthanasia or other borderline practices of medical behavior that potentially shorten life (MBPSL) and may be disguising problematic medical behavior. The Dutch figures on euthanasia and assisted suicide are reliant on self-reporting by physicians of their own medical behavior, which is why reporting has been such a big topic of concern by policymakers and researchers. Since the first quantitative data came out on euthanasia in The Netherlands in 1990, critics of the Dutch policy have rightly questioned whether evidence for the occurrence of a slippery slope is not hidden in other figures around MBPSL (Hendin 2002) and some have suggested that any MBPSL that includes an intention by the doctor to hasten death should be viewed as problematic (Hendin 2002:105). Proponents of the Dutch policy counter by suggesting that not all MBPSL are created equal (Pijnenborg and van der Maas 1993) and that intention is not a category of behavior by which MBPSL is legally weighed (Griffiths, et al. 2008:64). In addition, many MBPSL rates from The Netherlands are similar to rates found in other European countries, including rates of abstention, withdrawing or withholding treatments, pain relief with life shortening effects, and termination of life without the patient's explicit request for patients at the end of life who can no longer communicate and appear to be suffering severely (Griffiths, et al. 2008:158).

I believe that slippery slopes exist in medical practices at the end of life in countries with and without policies such as the *Termination of Life on Request and Assisted Suicide (Review Procedures) Act* (2002) in The Netherlands or the *Oregon Death with Dignity Act* (1997) in the U.S. Practices similar to euthanasia occur in places where it is not legal (Emanuel, et al. 2000; Heide, et al. 2003; Magnusson 2004; Meier, et al. 1998; Morita, et al. 2002) and borderline practices occur in places where euthanasia policies exist (Chabot 2007:158; Griffiths, et al. 2008). Chabot (2007), for instance, provides some evidence for borderline practices in his study of "auto-euthanasia," a term he uses to describe a type of suicide that occurs by patients mostly for medical reasons done in consultation with one or more persons, but without physician assistance or authorization. In each of these cases, an end-of-life association was consulted and patients died either by stopping eating and drinking or by lethal drug overdose. Looking at these cases, I believe that some (not all of them) could be categorized as suicide due to an over-integrated concept connecting infirmity with euthanasia (*altruistic*), a lack of cultural skills or ability to obtain legal euthanasia (*egoistic*), or suicide that falls outside of accepted norms and on the borderline of a slippery slope in effect in The Netherlands (*anomic*). In my study, I had several *huisartsen* report performing euthanasia prior to 1984 and had indication that terminal sedation was in use (see Chapter 4). As new medical behaviors that potentially shorten life emerge, such as terminal sedation or "auto-euthanasia", it is important that new regulations also emerge to adequately address these practices to ensure that they do not become practices that are used in lieu of regulated and professionally accepted forms of medical behavior.

Qualitative evidence from my study supports what we know from quantitative studies of euthanasia and other medical behaviors at the end of life (Onwuteaka-Philipsen, et al. 2007). When I looked closely at the talk that was occurring once a euthanasia request was made, I found patterns that suggest that once a patient initiates a request for euthanasia it is unlikely that euthanasia will occur without repeated and culturally-skilled effort on the part of the patient. Euthanasia talk progresses in stages and typically at the end of each stage the *huisarts* will pause discussions, leaving the patient confident that euthanasia death remains a viable option but without putting the patient in a position of not being able to stop this thing they have started. Patients who engage in euthanasia talk must also show some skill in how they engage in this discourse. Requests made in the absence of a terminal prognosis or requests made for reasons of psychological suffering were not favored by study *huisartsen*. Requests made by persons isolated from friends and family, by persons exhibiting untreatable depression, or by persons who were too pushy all gave study *huisartsen* reason to stall discussions. How euthanasia talk occurs in an acute care nursing facility with *verpleegartsen* or how it occurs in the Dutch hospital with specialists may differ, but in the homes and nursing homes I visited, *huisartsen* respond to these "red flags" by using the informal stages in euthanasia talk as places to slow down or stall progression towards euthanasia death.

My research finds that Foucauldian discourses like euthanasia talk do not provide all people equal access. While many may be familiar with this popular end-of-life discourse, not everyone will have the ability nor the inclination to engage in euthanasia talk the same way. My findings suggest the presence of mainstream activity around euthanasia talk, yet clearly demonstrate that there are individuals who fall outside of this mainstream. There are physicians who choose not to perform euthanasia and those who will do so under only the most extreme circumstances. There are patients who are not skilled in culturally-appropriate ways to ask for euthanasia or who choose not to participate based on religious or personal preferences. There are illnesses and conditions that are not favored by *huisartsen* who are considering a patient's request for euthanasia. Requests based on psychological suffering or requests with signs of depression, social isolation or unresolved family conflict give *huisartsen* reason to refuse to initiate euthanasia discussions or to stall euthanasia discussions begun under better circumstances. Likewise, requests for reasons of old age, tiredness with life, or diseases without a somewhat predictable trajectory of decline (such as heart disease) are not generally favored by *huisartsen* considering a patient's request for euthanasia.

Euthanasia for reasons of altruistic, egoistic or anomic suicide may well be occurring in The Netherlands, but my research and quantitative evidence suggest that for most patients euthanasia occurs as a discussion, rather than a life-ending act. Most of the people I spoke with did not want to die, but considered euthanasia as an ideal option in the event that their suffering became unmanageable. Euthanasia requests were not wishes for death, but more generally an insurance policy for the future.

Create Space for Processing Death and Invoking an Ideal

I opened this book with a story about a man who told me that a photograph was a better representation of his wife than the woman who lay dying in bed. When I watched my mother die, I saw for myself just what he meant. There is something about a person that can die prior to death of the body. Social death cannot be attributed to a single point in time, nor to a strict set of behaviors. It is a series of losses—lost identity and lost ability to participate in social activities and relationships—that eventually culminates in a perceived disconnection from social life. But even that is not absolute, no one participant may share the same perception toward a dying person and perceptions of social death may change in an instant with the re-occurrence of a smile or a glance taken to be meaningful.

Modern death is where sociality ends or is at least re-negotiated. Probably one of the more critical lessons that we can gain from this study is the importance of creating a space within the healthcare system for allowing patients, families, and practitioners to process what it means to die. In The Netherlands, space has been created in part within the existing structure of general practice and in larger form within the structure of euthanasia discussions. I watched many people die and before they died, I watched them live with all aspects of limitation and decline. With the advancements in medical knowledge and treatments, people are living longer with more chronic conditions. Not everyone I met experienced the same type or severity of loss, but for those who did lose the ability to participate in one or more daily activities, what they lost was more than simple physical comfort. These were social losses and these losses impacted on concepts of identity and self worth and on a person's ability to participate in relationships.

The Dutch response to social loss and social death has been to impart some order and control over the often chaotic and disorderly process of dying through euthanasia talk and euthanasia policy. As a society that favors the collective, it is a response based in dialogue among key participants and based in keeping even dying patients connected to their social networks for as long as possible. Euthanasia talk has evolved, in part, into a kind of palliative discourse in The Netherlands, helping patients and families negotiate in dialogue the transition from life to death. Through euthanasia talk, dying individuals and families assume active roles, they are empowered to make choices and decisions at the end of life, and they are able to process current circumstances in relation to a future ideal. This is just the kind of discourse that those who write about the importance of including spirituality in end-of-life care have been calling for (Baer 2001; Dossey 1993; Koenig and Lawson 2004; Puchalski 2006) and it is the kind of discourse that is sorely lacking in the American system of healthcare.

How ideal death is invoked in euthanasia talk is important. Ideal Dutch deaths are orderly; they are well discussed with family and the home healthcare team; they occur in a *gezellig* (warm, cozy) environment, typically at home and not in a hospital or institutional setting; they do not include excessive suffering; they leave good memories for surviving family; and the passing occurs surrounded by family and with support from Dutch home health care. When someone initiates euthanasia talk, they may well be initiating an attempt to control the timing of death to have death of the body more closely coincide with death of the social being (Seale 1998:183–191). More than that, however, there is something about having the possibility of an ideal death in front of a person that changes the present-day reality. Recall Mr. Veenstra's story from Chapter 6. His wife suffered for years with cancer, 10 months with a terminal prognosis and all sorts of bodily decline and social loss. Once they had finally decided on euthanasia, they still had to wait and suffer through another two weeks. Yet compared to his father's death, his wife's death was ideal. Both suffered many months prior to death and both received a lethal dose of medication to hasten death, but she had a euthanasia request and he did not. She and her family knew throughout her last months that if the worse came to bear that she had an option to end the suffering. This is something Mr. Veenstra's father did not have and something that most Americans do not have.

Clearly death and dying has changed in many places and so our responses to death must also change. Medicine has come to dominate end-of-life, largely overtaking religion at the bedside of the sick and the dying (Norwood 2006a). In places where medicine is prominent, it is important that discourses like euthanasia talk can exist within the medical structure. It does not necessarily need to be a discussion for planning a euthanasia death, but it needs to be some kind of dialogue within healthcare that invokes an ideal, whether these are options for comfort care, ceasing of futile treatments, or the option for some kind of assisted death. This kind of dialogue gives patients and families an ideal they can rely on during difficult stages of decline and they give health practitioners a role and a stake in helping create better deaths for their patients and their families.

Consider Assisted Dying in Cultural Context

Euthanasia as it is practiced in The Netherlands or elsewhere is a product of cultural process, so to critique or transfer such a policy it is important to take time to understand the cultural practices on which it based. My study reveals that when you look closely at the day-to-day practice of euthanasia, you find a practice that favors order, dialogue, compromise and faith in the collective to devise a process and a system that optimally cares for Dutch citizens. Euthanasia talk is a cultural construction based in a well-worn process of decision-making and conflict-resolution that the Dutch call *overleg*. The goal of euthanasia talk, like any good example of *overleg*, is not just about the end result (the death); it is about living the remainder of your life in ways that are Dutch familiar. *Overleg* provides the structure for processing end-of-life discussions and relies on input from all participants and an assurance that the rules for proper *overleg* are followed. In euthanasia talk, dying individuals discuss their request for euthanasia with family members and the *huisarts*, repeatedly talking about the reason for the request, allowing each participant equal time to weigh in about the request, and ultimately coming to a consensus with which all participants (*huisartsen*, patients and families) are comfortable. Individuals in The Netherlands have the right to choose euthanasia, but they do so within the context of input from family, who regularly participate in these dialogues, and physicians, who ultimately decide whether or not a euthanasia request can end in euthanasia death.

The U.S., on the other hand, does not have this emphasis on the collective, nor does it have these kind of pervasive cultural processes for mediating conflict in the doctor-patient-family relationship. Any policy to promote either euthanasia, or another type of discourse for invoking ideals and processing death, would in practice look quite different than the Dutch model. This is because in practice, we learn that policy conforms to what is culturally familiar.

Let us look at some of the cultural processes that are familiar in the U.S. In the U.S., our nation was founded on an ethic that set the development of the individual in conflict with authority and, not surprisingly, the U.S. system of healthcare is marked by a much more conflictive doctor-patient-family relationship. Ours is a system that favors individuals who fend for themselves over any type of comprehensive, state-supported system designed to offer assistance at the end of life. Thus any successful policy would take these and other central cultural processes into account.

Improving End-of-Life Care

In this book, I have introduced the idea that euthanasia is more often experienced as a discussion than as a life-ending act. This is an important shift in thinking about euthanasia that begs the question, just what are the Dutch talking about when they talk euthanasia? Looking closely at the day-to-day practice of euthanasia, I find both the obvious (that euthanasia talk is a discussion for the purpose of planning a euthanasia death) and the not so obvious (that it is a discussion that promotes social bonding and affirmation of life in the face of bodily decline, social loss and social death). In the first half of the book, I presented the contexts in which euthanasia and other medical behaviors at the end of life occur both in The Netherlands and the U.S. — from long-standing historical connections and developments to cultural characteristics that appear prominently at the end of Dutch and American life. I also introduce euthanasia as a type of Foucauldian discourse, a cultural form that encompasses and envelopes how people come to think, to feel and ultimately to act at the end of Dutch life. Foucault (1972; 1991) offers the framework for how to see past the obvious to the more subtle underpinnings of Dutch end of life practices and Seale (1998) offers clues to understanding the content of euthanasia talk, suggesting that end-of-life practices may well be a way the Dutch have developed to stave off social death.

In the second half of this book, I focused on the Dutch experience with euthanasia from the perspective of its three main participants in home death—*huisartsen*, patients and family members. For each group, I demonstrated how euthanasia talk works as a discourse and how social losses are managed through discussions that affirm sociality. For *huisartsen*, this meant having a presence at the end of life that does not necessarily revolve around treatment, but includes both guide and witness. It means invoking ideal concepts of death, falling back on constructions of the ideal in the event of difficult cases, and relying on shared cultural processes of decision-making to progress through and at times to stall euthanasia discussions. It also means a chance to deepen relationships with patients and family members, providing *huisartsen* the satisfaction of knowing that they are practitioners to the "whole" patient and their families through the life cycle from birth to death.

For patients, I demonstrated how euthanasia talk is used to invoke a future ideal death scenario that gives power to the dying individual in the present reality. It is also a way to exert control and order over bodily disruption, bridging present circumstances with a future ideal, giving space for processing meaning and reaffirming continuity in the face of disruption. Euthanasia talk helps maintain personhood in the face of decline, giving individuals an active role in scripting their own death and allowing for the active presence of Dutch society through the extensive system of home health care available in The Netherlands.

For families, I talked about how euthanasia talk provides family members a voice within healthcare that honors their central place in the life of the dying person and provides family members support within a cooperative relationship between family and state. Euthanasia talk gives families an ideal script for managing memories and family relationships in the face of losing a loved one. It gives some structure to families to process what it means to lose a family member and to come to new terms with various social losses and bodily indignities to which they are witness. Surviving family members are left to carry the memory of the life and the death of their loved one and, through euthanasia talk, Dutch society provides families with a space to re-work the memories they will carry based on ideal concepts of Dutch death.

Policy Implications

I subtitled this book, "lessons from The Netherlands," because I think that the Dutch experience offers important clues to how end-of-life care and policies can be improved, but only if this experience is understood in its proper context. Euthanasia, home care, general practice, healthcare and social safety nets in The Netherlands are all part of a system of long term and end-of-life care that is embedded in cultural form. Thus, *we first learn that policy is not transferable to other countries without consideration of both structural and cultural contexts.* Dutch welfare, healthcare, and euthanasia may not necessarily fit in other places without attention to what will and will not resonate with existing cultural norms and practices. The Netherlands has long supported a collective, welfare-model of government. The U.S., however, rose to power by questioning authority. A Puritan ethic laid the foundations for our nation, built on the rejection of both state and to some extent Church authority and based on a type of individualism where persons are encouraged to access the American dream according to their own devices and without government assistance. In practice, Dutch euthanasia policy emphasizes the role of the physician to administer lethal medication and the role of the collective (physicians, families and patients) to work in cooperation to process euthanasia talk. In U.S. healthcare, patients, families, and physicians have often been set in opposition to each other, as demonstrated by the patient's rights movement and the impact of malpractice in present-day medicine. It is not likely that a universal access model of healthcare that emphasizes coverage for all would resonate with the American people. It is also not likely that a euthanasia policy based on the physician's authority to decide euthanasia requests and administer lethal doses or euthanasia talk based in cooperative, discussion-based decision-making would fit in an American setting. What would fit in the U.S. today are the kind of policies that favor individual rights and choices. This means universal access in healthcare that provides an equitable level of care and support, but with the emphasis on individual choice. This also means a comprehensive system of end-of-life care that includes reforms to nursing home care, investment in home-based healthcare, continued attention on palliative care, and perhaps an assisted suicide policy that emphasizes the individual's right to choose—one choice among many real alternatives available to all persons at the end of life.

Second, good long term and end-of-life care includes supports and care that extends beyond medical concerns and treatments. Successful end-of-life care is so much more than the latest medical breakthroughs and treatments. It is about providing families with the supports they need to care for their loved ones and when family are not able to do that it is about stepping in to serve that function in the most humane and life-affirming way possible. Universal access to health and social supports is critical for transforming long term and end-of-life care in the U.S. American families are carrying too much of the burden and while gaps are sometimes filled locally by community- and faith-based organizations and in part by national programs of Medicare and Medicaid, this is not enough. Fixing this system does not necessarily mean spending more money on increasingly costly medical technologies, pharmaceuticals, or the latest medical advancements. It means spending wisely on home care, nursing and personal care, respite for families, and coordination of care, such as case management. It means doing further research on innovative and cost-effective solutions at the end of life, looking into new ways to allow citizens to remain in the community or new ways to structure nursing home care. It means tapping into local resources (community- and faith-based initiatives) that have come to find cost effective and humane, care-based programs for persons who are elderly, disabled or dying.

Finally, patients, families, and practitioners need space within the healthcare system where ideal death can be invoked to process what it means to die. As medicine has come to occupy the space surrounding death and dying, religion and religious rituals designed to allow dying individuals and their families time to process death have been displaced. People need time and space to process what it means to die well before death occurs. This is what helps them shape the meaning of the experience for those who are dying and for those who will survive. People need to be able to believe that there are options other than suffering at the end of life and they need to be able to invoke an ideal death to help manage the life that is remaining. Whether that means the option of assisted dying, clearer pathways for withdrawing and withholding futile treatments at the end of life, or a comprehensive system of palliative care for all persons regardless of ability to pay or some combination of these needs to be determined.

Too often, those who debate end-of-life policies have had too little information and have gotten bogged down in unresolved conflict where two sides talk at each other without hearing what the other has to offer. Both proponents and opponents of assisted dying in the U.S. have something important to say. Proponents of assisted dying in the U.S. show us some real shortfalls in our current system of end-of-life care and opponents offer important cautions about proceeding. It is my hope that the stories told in this book will give social scientists, healthcare professionals, families and policymakers more information to talk to each other and to find humane and caring ways to maintain life at the end of life.

List of Expert Interviews

In addition to interviews and observation, with *huisartsen*, their patients and their patients' families, I conducted interviews or consulted with experts on the place of euthanasia in broader social, cultural and religious context with the following persons. Interviews with these persons shaped the analysis, but no person listed below is responsible for the conclusions drawn in this ethnographic study.

American Anthropological Association, annual meeting presentation, Washington, DC 2001

American Anthropological Association, annual meeting presentation, San Jose, California, 2006

Amsterdam Thuiszorg employees, Amsterdam

Margaret P. Battin, PhD, bioethicist, University of Utah, Salt Lake City, Utah

Willem Beertse, *Uitvaartcentrum Zuid*, Amsterdam

Sander Borgsteede, PhD, *Free University,* Amsterdam

Diny de Bresser, Group Director, *Amsterdam Thuiszorg*, Amsterdam

Boudewijn Chabot, MD, Haarlem

Dirk van Dijk, *Amsterdam Thuiszorg*, Amsterdam

Anneke Frank, Rio (on home care coordination), Amstelveen

Free University, Department of Social Medicine symposium presentation, Amsterdam, 2001

Sjaak van der Geest, PhD, anthropologist, *Department of Anthropology, University of Amsterdam,* Amsterdam

A.J. Gelderblom, PhD, *Department of Literature, Utrecht University*, Utrecht

Peter Goodwin, MD, *Compassion & Choices,* Portland, Oregon

John Griffiths, PhD, sociologist of law, *University of Groningen*, Groningen

Tony Hak, PhD, medical sociologist, *Department of Social Medicine, Free University*, Amsterdam

Larry Heintz, PhD, philosopher and medical ethics, *University of Hawaii*, Hawaii

Caroline van der Horst, chaplain, *Sint Jacob*, Amsterdam

Linda F. Hogle, PhD, medical anthropologist, *University of Wisconsin, School of Medicine, Department of Medical History and Bioethics*, Madison, Wisconsin

Marijke der Horst, *Hospice Kuria*, Amsterdam

Dr. Jochemsen, *Prof. G.A. Lindeboom Instituut*, Ede

C. Kalis, *R.K. Begraafplaats Buitenveldert*, Amsterdam

James Kennedy, PhD, historian, *Hope College*, Holland, Michigan

Gerrit Kimsma, MD, M.Ph., bioethicist, *Free University*, Amsterdam

Albert Klijn, PhD, socio-legal researcher, *Ministry of Justice (WODC)*, Den Haag

Roel de Leeuw, *Nederlandse Vereniging voor Vrijwillige Euthanasie*, Amsterdam

Evert van Leeuwen, PhD, bioethicist, *Free University*, Amsterdam

Ellen Looman, humanistic chaplain, *de Venser*, Amsterdam

David Mehr, MD, *University of Missouri*, Columbia, Missouri

Bregje Onwuteaka-Philipsen, MA, PhD, *Department of Social Medicine, Free University*, Amsterdam

Henk Poolen, *Terra Nova Uitvaartvereniging*, Utrecht

Marijaane van der Schalk, MD, palliative care specialist and verpleegarts, *Sint Jacob*, Amsterdam

Piet Schoonheim, MD, huisarts trainer, *Free University*, Amsterdam

Promotie Club, University of Amsterdam, Medische Antropologie, Amsterdam

SISWO (Social Science and Health Issues) Symposium presentation, *University of Amsterdam*, Amsterdam, 2001

Stichting SOKA, De Regie over het Leven, Cure & Care conference, September 29, 2001

Anne-Mei The, PhD, medical anthropologist, *Department of Social Medicine, Free University*, Amsterdam

Dr. J van der Ven, PhD, theologian, *Katholieke Universiteit*, Nijmegen

Raymond de Vries, PhD, medical sociologist, *Bioethics Program, University of Michigan School of Medicine,* Ann Arbor, MI

Gerrit van der Wal, MD, PhD, chair, *Department of Social Medicine, Free University,* Amsterdam

Marjan Westerman, PhD, *Department of Social Medicine, Free University,* Amsterdam

Dick Willems, MD, PhD, bioethicist, *Department of Social Medicine, Vrije Univesiteit,* Amsterdam

Dutch Termination of Life on Request and Assisted Suicide (Review Procedures) Act (2002)

Termination of Life on Request and
Assisted Suicide (Review Procedures) Act
— This Act entered into force on April 1, 2002 —

Review procedures of termination of life on request and assisted suicide and amendment to the Penal Code (Wetboek van Strafrecht) and the Burial and Cremation Act (Wet op de lijkbezorging)

We Beatrix, by the grace of God, Queen of The Netherlands, Princess of Oranje-Nassau, etc., etc., etc.

Greetings to all who shall see or hear these presents! Be it known: Whereas We have considered that it is desired to include a ground for exemption from criminal liability for the physician who with due observance of the requirements of due care to be laid down by law terminates a life on request or assists in a suicide of another person, and to provide a statutory notification and review procedure; We, therefore, having heard the Council of State, and in consultation with the States General, have approved and decreed as We hereby approve and decree:

Chapter I. Definitions of Terms

Article 1
For the purposes of this Act:

a. Our Ministers mean the Ministers of Justice and of Health, Welfare and Sports;

b. assisted suicide means intentionally assisting in a suicide of another person or procuring for that other person the means referred to in Article 294 second paragraph, second sentence of the Penal code;

c. the physician means the physician who according to the notification has terminated a life on request or assisted in a suicide;

d. the consultant means the physician who has been consulted with respect to the intention by the physician to terminate a life on request or to assist in a suicide;

e. the providers of care mean the providers of care referred to in Article 446 first paragraph of Book 7 of the Civil Code (Burgerlijk Wetboek);

f. the committee means a regional review committee referred to in Article 3;

g. the regional inspector means the regional inspector of the Health Care Inspectorate of the Public Health Supervisory Service.

Chapter II. Requirements of Due Care

Article 2

1. The requirements of due care, referred to in Article 293 second paragraph Penal Code mean that the physician:

a. holds the conviction that the request by the patient was voluntary and well-considered,

b. holds the conviction that the patient's suffering was lasting and unbearable,

c. has informed the patient about the situation he was in and about his prospects,

d. and the patient hold the conviction that there was no other reasonable solution for the situation he was in,

e. has consulted at least one other, independent physician who has seen the patient and has given his written opinion on the requirements of due care, referred to in parts a–d, and

f. has terminated a life or assisted in a suicide with due care.

2. If the patient aged sixteen years or older is no longer capable of expressing his will, but prior to reaching this condition was deemed to have a reasonable understanding of his interests and has made a written statement containing a request for termination of life, the physician may carry out this request. The requirements of due care, referred to in the first paragraph, apply mutatis mutandis.

3. If the minor patient has attained an age between sixteen and eighteen years and may be deemed to have a reasonable understanding of his interests, the physician may carry out the patient's request for termination of life or assisted suicide, after the parent or the parents exercising parental authority and/or his guardian have been involved in the decision process.

4. If the minor patient is aged between twelve and sixteen years and may be deemed to have a reasonable understanding of his interests, the physician may carry out the patient's request, provided always that the parent or the parents exercising parental authority and/or his guardian agree with the termination of life or the assisted suicide. The second paragraph applies mutatis mutandis.

Chapter Ill. The Regional Review Committees for Termination of Life on Request and Assisted Suicide.

Paragraph 1: Establishment, composition and appointment
Article 3

1. There are regional committees for the review of notifications of cases of termination of life on request and assistance in a suicide as referred to in Article 293 second paragraph or 294 second paragraph second sentence, respectively, of the Penal Code.

2. A committee is composed of an uneven number of members, including at any rate one legal specialist, also chairman, one physician and one expert on ethical or philosophical issues'. The

committee also contains deputy members of each of the, categories listed in the first sentence.

Article 4

1. The chairman and the members, as well as the deputy members are appointed by Our Ministers for a period of six years. They may be re-appointed one time for another period of six years. 'philosophical issues'—in the original text the Dutch word 'zingevingsvraagstukken' is used to describe the discussion on the prerequisites for a meaningful life.

2. A committee has a secretary and one or more deputy secretaries, all legal specialists, appointed by Our Ministers. The secretary has an advisory role in the committee meetings.

3. The secretary may solely be held accountable by the committee for his activities for the committee.

Paragraph 2: Dismissal

Article 5

Our Ministers may at any time dismiss the chairman and the members, as well as the deputy members at their own request.

Article 6

Our Ministers may dismiss the chairman and the members, as well as the deputy members for reasons of unsuitability or incompetence or for other important reasons.

Paragraph 3: Remuneration

Article 7

The chairman and the members, as well as the deputy members receive a holiday allowance as well as a reimbursement of the travel and accommodation expenses according to the existing government scheme insofar as these expenses are not otherwise reimbursed from the State Funds.

Paragraph 4: Duties and powers

Article 8

1. The committee assesses on the basis of the report referred to in Article 7 second paragraph of the Burial and Cremation Act whether the physician who has terminated a life on request or assisted in a suicide has acted in accordance with the requirements of due care, referred to in Article 2.

2. The committee may request the physician to supplement his report in writing or verbally, where this is necessary for a proper assessment of the physician's actions.

3. The committee may make enquiries at the municipal autopsist, the consultant or the providers of care involved where this is necessary for a proper assessment of the physician's actions.

Article 9

1. The committee informs the physician within six weeks of the receipt of the report referred to in Article 8 first paragraph in writing of its motivated opinion.

2. The committee informs the Board of Procurators General and the regional health care inspector of its opinion:

> a. if the committee is of the opinion that the physician has failed to act in accordance with the requirements of due care, referred to in Article 2; or
>
> b. if a situation occurs as referred to in Article 12, final sentence of the Burial and Cremation Act.

The committee shall inform the physician of this.

3. The term referred to in the first paragraph may be extended one time by a maximum period of six weeks. The committee shall inform the physician of this.

4. The committee may provide a further, verbal explanation on its opinion to the physician. This verbal explanation may take place at the request of the committee or at the request of the physician.

Article 10

The committee is obliged to provide all information to the public prosecutor, at his request, which he may need:

> 1. for the benefit of the assessment of the physician's actions in the case referred to in Article 9 second paragraph;or
>
> 2. for the benefit of a criminal investigation.

The committee shall inform the physician of any provision of information to the public prosecutor.

Paragraph 6: Working method

Article 11

The committee shall ensure the registration of the cases of termination of life or assisted suicide reported for assessment. Further rules on this may be laid down by a ministerial regulation by Our Ministers.

Article 12

1. An opinion is adopted by a simple majority of votes.

2. An opinion may only be adopted by the committee provided all committee members have participated in the vote.

Article 13

At least twice a year, the chairmen of the regional review committees conduct consultations with one another with respect to the working method and the performance of the committees. A representative of the Board of Procurators General and a representative of the Health Care Inspectorate of the Public Health Supervisory Service are invited to attend these consultations.

Paragraph 7: Secrecy and Exemption

Article 14

The members and deputy members of the committee are under an obligation of secrecy to keep confidential any information acquired in the performance of their duties, except where any statutory regulation obliges them to divulge this information or where the necessity to divulge information ensues from their duties.

Article 15

A member of the committee that serves on the committee in the treatment of a case exempts himself and may be challenged if there are facts or circumstances that may affect the impartiality of his opinion.

Article 16

A member, a deputy member and the secretary of the committee refrain from rendering an opinion on the intention by a physician to terminate a life on request or to assist in a suicide.

Paragraph 8: Report

Article 17

1. Not later than 1 April, the committees issue a joint annual report to Our Ministers on the activities of the past calendar year. Our Ministers shall lay down a model for this by means of a ministerial regulation.

2. The report on the activities referred to in the first paragraph shall at any rate include the following:

    a. the number of reported cases of termination of life on request and assisted suicide on which the committee has rendered an opinion;

    b. the nature of these cases;

    c. the opinions and the considerations involved.

Article 18

Annually, at the occasion of the submission of the budget to the States General, Our Ministers shall issue a report with respect to the performance of the committees further to the report on the activities as referred to in Article 17 first paragraph.

Article 19

1. On the recommendation of Our Ministers, rules shall be laid down by order in council regarding the committees with respect to

    a. their number and their territorial jurisdiction;

    b. their domicile.

2. Our Ministers may lay down further rules by or pursuant to an order in council regarding the committees with respect to

    a. their size and composition;

    b. their working method and reports.

Chapter IV. Amendments to other Acts

Article 20

The Penal Code shall be amended as follows:

A

Article 293 shall read:

Article 293

1. Any person who terminates another person's life at that person's express and earnest request shall be liable to a term of imprisonment not exceeding twelve years or a fifth-category fine.

2. The act referred to in the first paragraph shall not be an offence if it committed by a physician who fulfils the due care criteria set out in Article 2 of the Termination of Life on Request and Assisted Suicide (Review Procedures) Act, and if the

physician notifies the municipal pathologist of this act in accordance with the provisions of Article 7, paragraph 2 of the Burial and Cremation Act.

B

Article 294 shall read:

Article 294

1. Any person who intentionally incites another to commit suicide shall, if suicide follows, be liable to a term of imprisonment not exceeding three years or a fine of the fourth-category fine.

2. Any person who intentionally assists another to commit suicide or provides him with the means to do so shall, if suicide follows, be liable to a term of imprisonment not exceeding three years or a fourth-category fine. Article 293, paragraph 2 shall apply mutatis mutandis.

C

In Article 295, the following is inserted after '293': first paragraph.

D

In Article 422, the following is inserted after '293': first paragraph.

Article 21

The Burial and Cremation Act shall be amended as follows:

A

Article 7 shall read:

Article 7

1. A person who has performed a postmortem shall issue a death certificate if he is convinced that death has occurred as a result of a natural cause.

2. If the death was the result of the application of termination of life on request or assisted suicide as referred to in Article 293 second paragraph or Article 294 second paragraph second sentence, respectively, of the Penal Code, the attending physician shall not issue a death certificate and shall promptly notify the municipal autopsist or one of the municipal autopsists of the cause of death by completing a form. The physician shall supplement this form with a reasoned report with respect to the due observance of the requirements of due care referred to in

Article 2 of the Termination of Life on Request and Assisted Suicide (Review Procedures) act.

3. If the attending physician in other cases than referred to in the second paragraph believes that he may not issue a death certificate, he must promptly notify the municipal autopsist or one of the municipal autopsists of this by completing a form.

B

Article 9 shall read:

Article 9

1. The form and the set-up of the models of the death certificate to be issued by the attending physician and by the municipal autopsist shall be laid down by order in council.

2. The form and the set-up of the models of the notification and the report referred to in Article 7 second paragraph, of the notification referred to in Article 7 third paragraph and of the forms referred to in Article 10 first and second paragraph shall be laid down by order in council on the recommendation of Our Minister of Justice and Our Minister of Health, Welfare and Sports.

C

Article 10 shall read:

Article 10

1. If the municipal autopsist is of the opinion that he cannot issue a death certificate, he shall promptly report this to the public prosecutor by completing a form and he shall promptly notify the registrar of births, deaths and marriages.

2. In the event of a notification as referred to in Article 7 second paragraph and without prejudice to the first paragraph, the municipal autopsist shall promptly report to the regional review committee referred to in Article 3 of the Termination of Life on Request and Assisted Suicide (Review Procedures) Act by completing a form. He shall enclose a reasoned report as referred to in Article 7 second paragraph.

D

The following sentence shall be added to Article 12, reading: If the public prosecutor, in the cases referred to in Article 7 second paragraph, is of the opinion that he cannot issue a certificate of no objection against the burial or cremation, he shall promptly inform the municipal autopsist and the regional review committee referred to in Article 3 of the Termination of Life on Request and Assisted Suicide (Review Procedures) Act of this.

E

In Article 81, first part, '7, first paragraph' shall be replaced by '7, first and second paragraph'.

Article 22

The General Administrative Law Act (Algemene wet bestuursrecht) shall be amended as follows:

At the end of part d of Article 1:6, the full stop shall be replaced by a semicolon and the following shall be added to the fifth part, reading:

> e. decisions and actions in the implementation of the Termination of Life and Assisted Suicide (Review Procedures) Act.

Chapter V. Final Provisions

Article 23

This Act shall take effect as of a date to be determined by Royal Decree.

Article 24

This Act may be cited as: Termination of Life on Request and Assisted Suicide (Review Procedures) Act.

We hereby order and command that this Act shall be published in the Bulletin of Acts and Decrees and that all ministerial departments, authorities, bodies and officials whom it may concern shall diligently implement it.

Done

The Minister of Justice,

The Minister of Health, Welfare and Sports.

Upper House, parliamentary year 2000–2001, 26 691, no 137

Oregon Death with Dignity Act (1997)

THE OREGON DEATH WITH DIGNITY ACT
OREGON REVISED STATUTES

(General Provisions)

(Section 1)

Note: The division headings, subdivision headings and leadlines for 127.800 to 127.890, 127.895 and 127.897 were enacted as part of Ballot Measure 16 (1994) and were not provided by Legislative Counsel.

127.800 §1.01. Definitions. The following words and phrases, whenever used in ORS 127.800 to 127.897, have the following meanings:

(1) "Adult" means an individual who is 18 years of age or older.

(2) "Attending physician" means the physician who has primary responsibility for the care of the patient and treatment of the patient's terminal disease.

(3) "Capable" means that in the opinion of a court or in the opinion of the patient's attending physician or consulting physician, psychiatrist or psychologist, a patient has the ability to make and communicate health care decisions to health care providers, including communication through persons familiar with the patient's manner of communicating if those persons are available.

(4) "Consulting physician" means a physician who is qualified by specialty or experience to make a professional diagnosis and prognosis regarding the patient's disease.

(5) "Counseling" means one or more consultations as necessary between a state licensed psychiatrist or psychologist and a patient for the purpose of determining that the patient is capable and not suffering from a psychiatric or psychological disorder or depression causing impaired judgment.

(6) "Health care provider" means a person licensed, certified or otherwise authorized or permitted by the law of this state to administer health care or dispense medication in the ordinary course of business or practice of a profession, and includes a health care facility.

(7) "Informed decision" means a decision by a qualified patient, to request and obtain a prescription to end his or her life in a humane and dignified manner, that is based on an appreciation of the relevant facts and after being fully informed by the attending physician of:

(a) His or her medical diagnosis;

(b) His or her prognosis;

(c) The potential risks associated with taking the medication to be prescribed;

(d) The probable result of taking the medication to be prescribed; and

(e) The feasible alternatives, including, but not limited to, comfort care, hospice care and pain control.

(8) "Medically confirmed" means the medical opinion of the attending physician has been confirmed by a consulting physician who has examined the patient and the patient's relevant medical records.

(9) "Patient" means a person who is under the care of a physician.

(10) "Physician" means a doctor of medicine or osteopathy licensed to practice medicine by the Board of Medical Examiners for the State of Oregon.

(11) "Qualified patient" means a capable adult who is a resident of Oregon and has satisfied the requirements of ORS 127.800 to 127.897 in order to obtain a prescription for medication to end his or her life in a humane and dignified manner.

(12) "Terminal disease" means an incurable and irreversible disease that has been medically confirmed and will, within reasonable

medical judgment, produce death within six months. [1995 c.3 §1.01; 1999 c.423 §1]
(Written Request for Medication to End One's Life in a Humane and Dignified Manner)
(Section 2)
127.805 §2.01. Who may initiate a written request for medication. (1) An adult who is capable, is a resident of Oregon, and has been determined by the attending physician and consulting physician to be suffering from a terminal disease, and who has voluntarily expressed his or her wish to die, may make a written request for medication for the purpose of ending his or her life in a humane and dignified manner in accordance with ORS 127.800 to 127.897.

(2) No person shall qualify under the provisions of ORS 127.800 to 127.897 solely because of age or disability. [1995 c.3 §2.01; 1999 c.423 §2]

127.810 §2.02. Form of the written request. (1) A valid request for medication under ORS 127.800 to 127.897 shall be in substantially the form described in ORS 127.897, signed and dated by the patient and witnessed by at least two individuals who, in the presence of the patient, attest that to the best of their knowledge and belief the patient is capable, acting voluntarily, and is not being coerced to sign the request.

(2) One of the witnesses shall be a person who is not:

(a) A relative of the patient by blood, marriage or adoption;

(b) A person who at the time the request is signed would be entitled to any portion of the estate of the qualified patient upon death under any will or by operation of law; or

(c) An owner, operator or employee of a health care facility where the qualified patient is receiving medical treatment or is a resident.

(3) The patient's attending physician at the time the request is signed shall not be a witness.

(4) If the patient is a patient in a long term care facility at the time the written request is made, one of the witnesses shall be an individual designated by the facility and having the qualifications specified by the Department of Human Services by rule. [1995 c.3 §2.02]

(Safeguards)

(Section 3)

127.815 §3.01. Attending physician responsibilities. (1) The attending physician shall:

(a) Make the initial determination of whether a patient has a terminal disease, is capable, and has made the request voluntarily;

(b) Request that the patient demonstrate Oregon residency pursuant to ORS 127.860;

(c) To ensure that the patient is making an informed decision, inform the patient of:

(A) His or her medical diagnosis;

(B) His or her prognosis;

(C) The potential risks associated with taking the medication to be prescribed;

(D) The probable result of taking the medication to be prescribed; and

(E) The feasible alternatives, including, but not limited to, comfort care, hospice care and pain control;

(d) Refer the patient to a consulting physician for medical confirmation of the diagnosis, and for a determination that the patient is capable and acting voluntarily;

(e) Refer the patient for counseling if appropriate pursuant to ORS 127.825;

(f) Recommend that the patient notify next of kin;

(g) Counsel the patient about the importance of having another person present when the patient takes the medication prescribed pursuant to ORS 127.800 to 127.897 and of not taking the medication in a public place;

(h) Inform the patient that he or she has an opportunity to rescind the request at any time and in any manner, and offer the patient an opportunity to rescind at the end of the 15 day waiting period pursuant to ORS 127.840;

(i) Verify, immediately prior to writing the prescription for medication under ORS 127.800 to 127.897, that the patient is making an informed decision;

(j) Fulfill the medical record documentation requirements of ORS 127.855;

(k) Ensure that all appropriate steps are carried out in accordance with ORS 127.800 to 127.897 prior to writing a prescription for medication to enable a qualified patient to end his or her life in a humane and dignified manner; and

(L)(A) Dispense medications directly, including ancillary medications intended to facilitate the desired effect to minimize the patient's discomfort, provided the attending physician is registered as a dispensing physician with the Board of Medical Examiners, has a current Drug Enforcement Administration certificate and complies with any applicable administrative rule; or

(B) With the patient's written consent:

(i) Contact a pharmacist and inform the pharmacist of the prescription; and

(ii) Deliver the written prescription personally or by mail to the pharmacist, who will dispense the medications to either the patient, the attending physician or an expressly identified agent of the patient.

(2) Notwithstanding any other provision of law, the attending physician may sign the patient's death certificate. [1995 c.3 §3.01; 1999 c.423 §3]

127.820 §3.02. Consulting physician confirmation. Before a patient is qualified under ORS 127.800 to 127.897, a consulting physician shall examine the patient and his or her relevant medical records and confirm, in writing, the attending physician's diagnosis that the patient is suffering from a terminal disease, and verify that the patient is capable, is acting voluntarily and has made an informed decision. [1995 c.3 §3.02]

127.825 §3.03. Counseling referral. If in the opinion of the attending physician or the consulting physician a patient may be suffering from a psychiatric or psychological disorder or depression causing impaired judgment, either physician shall refer the patient for counseling. No medication to end a patient's life in a humane and dignified manner shall be prescribed until the person performing the counseling determines that the patient is not suffering from a psychiatric or psychological disorder or depression causing impaired judgment. [1995 c.3 §3.03; 1999 c.423 §4]

127.830 §3.04. Informed decision. No person shall receive a prescription for medication to end his or her life in a humane and dignified manner unless he or she has made an informed decision as defined in ORS 127.800 (7). Immediately prior to writing a prescription for medication under ORS 127.800 to 127.897, the attending physician shall verify that the patient is making an informed decision. [1995 c.3 §3.04]

127.835 §3.05. Family notification. The attending physician shall recommend that the patient notify the next of kin of his or her request for medication pursuant to ORS 127.800 to 127.897. A patient who declines or is unable to notify next of kin shall not have his or her request denied for that reason. [1995 c.3 §3.05; 1999 c.423 §6]

127.840 §3.06. Written and oral requests. In order to receive a prescription for medication to end his or her life in a humane and dignified manner, a qualified patient shall have made an oral request and a written request, and reiterate the oral request to his or her attending physician no less than fifteen (15) days after making the initial oral request. At the time the qualified patient makes his or her second oral request, the attending physician shall offer the patient an opportunity to rescind the request. [1995 c.3 §3.06]

127.845 §3.07. Right to rescind request. A patient may rescind his or her request at any time and in any manner without regard to his or her mental state. No prescription for medication under ORS 127.800 to 127.897 may be written without the attending physician offering the qualified patient an opportunity to rescind the request. [1995 c.3 §3.07]

127.850 §3.08. Waiting periods. No less than fifteen (15) days shall elapse between the patient's initial oral request and the writing of a prescription under ORS 127.800 to 127.897. No less than 48 hours shall elapse between the patient's written request and the writing of a prescription under ORS 127.800 to 127.897. [1995 c.3 §3.08]

127.855 §3.09. Medical record documentation requirements. The following shall be documented or filed in the patient's medical record:

(1) All oral requests by a patient for medication to end his or her life in a humane and dignified manner;

(2) All written requests by a patient for medication to end his or her life in a humane and dignified manner;

(3) The attending physician's diagnosis and prognosis, determination that the patient is capable, acting voluntarily and has made an informed decision;

(4) The consulting physician's diagnosis and prognosis, and verification that the patient is capable, acting voluntarily and has made an informed decision;

(5) A report of the outcome and determinations made during counseling, if performed;

(6) The attending physician's offer to the patient to rescind his or her request at the time of the patient's second oral request pursuant to ORS 127.840; and

(7) A note by the attending physician indicating that all requirements under ORS 127.800 to 127.897 have been met and indicating the steps taken to carry out the request, including a notation of the medication prescribed. [1995 c.3 §3.09]

127.860 §3.10. Residency requirement. Only requests made by Oregon residents under ORS 127.800 to 127.897 shall be granted. Factors demonstrating Oregon residency include but are not limited to:

(1) Possession of an Oregon driver license;

(2) Registration to vote in Oregon;

(3) Evidence that the person owns or leases property in Oregon; or

(4) Filing of an Oregon tax return for the most recent tax year. [1995 c.3 §3.10; 1999 c.423 §8]

127.865 §3.11. Reporting requirements. (1)(a) The Department of Human Services shall annually review a sample of records maintained pursuant to ORS 127.800 to 127.897.

(b) The department shall require any health care provider upon dispensing medication pursuant to ORS 127.800 to 127.897 to file a copy of the dispensing record with the department.

(2) The department shall make rules to facilitate the collection of information regarding compliance with ORS 127.800 to 127.897. Ex-

cept as otherwise required by law, the information collected shall not be a public record and may not be made available for inspection by the public.

(3) The department shall generate and make available to the public an annual statistical report of information collected under subsection (2) of this section. [1995 c.3 §3.11; 1999 c.423 §9; 2001 c.104 §40]

127.870 §3.12. Effect on construction of wills, contracts and statutes. (1) No provision in a contract, will or other agreement, whether written or oral, to the extent the provision would affect whether a person may make or rescind a request for medication to end his or her life in a humane and dignified manner, shall be valid.

(2) No obligation owing under any currently existing contract shall be conditioned or affected by the making or rescinding of a request, by a person, for medication to end his or her life in a humane and dignified manner. [1995 c.3 §3.12]

127.875 §3.13. Insurance or annuity policies. The sale, procurement, or issuance of any life, health, or accident insurance or annuity policy or the rate charged for any policy shall not be conditioned upon or affected by the making or rescinding of a request, by a person, for medication to end his or her life in a humane and dignified manner. Neither shall a qualified patient's act of ingesting medication to end his or her life in a humane and dignified manner have an effect upon a life, health, or accident insurance or annuity policy. [1995 c.3 §3.13]

127.880 §3.14. Construction of Act. Nothing in ORS 127.800 to 127.897 shall be construed to authorize a physician or any other person to end a patient's life by lethal injection, mercy killing or active euthanasia. Actions taken in accordance with ORS 127.800 to 127.897 shall not, for any purpose, constitute suicide, assisted suicide, mercy killing or homicide, under the law. [1995 c.3 §3.14]

(Immunities and Liabilities)

(Section 4)

127.885 §4.01. Immunities; basis for prohibiting health care provider from participation; notification; permissible sanctions. Except as provided in ORS 127.890:

(1) No person shall be subject to civil or criminal liability or professional disciplinary action for participating in good faith compliance with ORS 127.800 to 127.897. This includes being present when a qualified patient takes the prescribed medication to end his or her life in a humane and dignified manner.

(2) No professional organization or association, or health care provider, may subject a person to censure, discipline, suspension, loss of license, loss of privileges, loss of membership or other penalty for participating or refusing to participate in good faith compliance with ORS 127.800 to 127.897.

(3) No request by a patient for or provision by an attending physician of medication in good faith compliance with the provisions of ORS 127.800 to 127.897 shall constitute neglect for any purpose of law or provide the sole basis for the appointment of a guardian or conservator.

(4) No health care provider shall be under any duty, whether by contract, by statute or by any other legal requirement to participate in the provision to a qualified patient of medication to end his or her life in a humane and dignified manner. If a health care provider is unable or unwilling to carry out a patient's request under ORS 127.800 to 127.897, and the patient transfers his or her care to a new health care provider, the prior health care provider shall transfer, upon request, a copy of the patient's relevant medical records to the new health care provider.

(5)(a) Notwithstanding any other provision of law, a health care provider may prohibit another health care provider from participating in ORS 127.800 to 127.897 on the premises of the prohibiting provider if the prohibiting provider has notified the health care provider of the prohibiting provider's policy regarding participating in ORS 127.800 to 127.897. Nothing in this paragraph prevents a health care provider from providing health care services to a patient that do not constitute participation in ORS 127.800 to 127.897.

(b) Notwithstanding the provisions of subsections (1) to (4) of this section, a health care provider may subject another health care provider to the sanctions stated in this paragraph if the sanctioning health care provider has notified the sanctioned provider prior to participation in ORS 127.800 to 127.897 that it prohibits participation in ORS 127.800 to 127.897:

(A) Loss of privileges, loss of membership or other sanction provided pursuant to the medical staff bylaws, policies and procedures of the sanctioning health care provider if the sanctioned provider is a member of the sanctioning provider's medical staff and participates in ORS 127.800 to 127.897 while on the health care facility premises, as defined in ORS 442.015, of the sanctioning health care provider, but not including the private medical office of a physician or other provider;

(B) Termination of lease or other property contract or other nonmonetary remedies provided by lease contract, not including loss or restriction of medical staff privileges or exclusion from a provider panel, if the sanctioned provider participates in ORS 127.800 to 127.897 while on the premises of the sanctioning health care provider or on property that is owned by or under the direct control of the sanctioning health care provider; or

(C) Termination of contract or other nonmonetary remedies provided by contract if the sanctioned provider participates in ORS 127.800 to 127.897 while acting in the course and scope of the sanctioned provider's capacity as an employee or independent contractor of the sanctioning health care provider. Nothing in this subparagraph shall be construed to prevent:

(i) A health care provider from participating in ORS 127.800 to 127.897 while acting outside the course and scope of the provider's capacity as an employee or independent contractor; or

(ii) A patient from contracting with his or her attending physician and consulting physician to act outside the course and scope of the provider's capacity as an employee or independent contractor of the sanctioning health care provider.

(c) A health care provider that imposes sanctions pursuant to paragraph (b) of this subsection must follow all due process and other procedures the sanctioning health care provider may have that are related to the imposition of sanctions on another health care provider.

(d) For purposes of this subsection:

(A) "Notify" means a separate statement in writing to the health care provider specifically informing the health care provider prior to the provider's participation in ORS 127.800 to 127.897 of the sanctioning health care provider's policy about participation in activities covered by ORS 127.800 to 127.897.

(B) "Participate in ORS 127.800 to 127.897" means to perform the duties of an attending physician pursuant to ORS 127.815, the consulting physician function pursuant to ORS 127.820 or the counseling function pursuant to ORS 127.825. "Participate in ORS 127.800 to 127.897" does not include:

(i) Making an initial determination that a patient has a terminal disease and informing the patient of the medical prognosis;

(ii) Providing information about the Oregon Death with Dignity Act to a patient upon the request of the patient;

(iii) Providing a patient, upon the request of the patient, with a referral to another physician; or

(iv) A patient contracting with his or her attending physician and consulting physician to act outside of the course and scope of the provider's capacity as an employee or independent contractor of the sanctioning health care provider.

(6) Suspension or termination of staff membership or privileges under subsection (5) of this section is not reportable under ORS 441.820. Action taken pursuant to ORS 127.810, 127.815, 127.820 or 127.825 shall not be the sole basis for a report of unprofessional or dishonorable conduct under ORS 677.415 (2) or (3).

(7) No provision of ORS 127.800 to 127.897 shall be construed to allow a lower standard of care for patients in the community where the patient is treated or a similar community. [1995 c.3 §4.01; 1999 c.423 §10]

Note: As originally enacted by the people, the leadline to section 4.01 read "Immunities." The remainder of the leadline was added by editorial action.

127.890 §4.02. Liabilities. (1) A person who without authorization of the patient willfully alters or forges a request for medication or conceals or destroys a rescission of that request with the intent or effect of causing the patient's death shall be guilty of a Class A felony.

(2) A person who coerces or exerts undue influence on a patient to request medication for the purpose of ending the patient's life, or to destroy a rescission of such a request, shall be guilty of a Class A felony.

(3) Nothing in ORS 127.800 to 127.897 limits further liability for civil damages resulting from other negligent conduct or intentional misconduct by any person.

(4) The penalties in ORS 127.800 to 127.897 do not preclude criminal penalties applicable under other law for conduct which is inconsistent with the provisions of ORS 127.800 to 127.897. [1995 c.3 §4.02]

127.892 Claims by governmental entity for costs incurred. Any governmental entity that incurs costs resulting from a person terminating his or her life pursuant to the provisions of ORS 127.800 to 127.897 in a public place shall have a claim against the estate of the person to recover such costs and reasonable attorney fees related to enforcing the claim. [1999 c.423 §5a]

(Severability)

(Section 5)

127.895 §5.01. Severability. Any section of ORS 127.800 to 127.897 being held invalid as to any person or circumstance shall not affect the application of any other section of ORS 127.800 to 127.897 which can be given full effect without the invalid section or application. [1995 c.3 §5.01]

(Form of the Request)

(Section 6)

127.897 §6.01. Form of the request. A request for a medication as authorized by ORS 127.800 to 127.897 shall be in substantially the following form:

REQUEST FOR MEDICATION
TO END MY LIFE IN A HUMANE
AND DIGNIFIED MANNER

I, _____, am an adult of sound mind.
I am suffering from _____, which my attending physician has determined is a terminal disease and which has been medically confirmed by a consulting physician.

I have been fully informed of my diagnosis, prognosis, the nature of medication to be prescribed and potential associated risks, the expected result, and the feasible alternatives, including comfort care, hospice care and pain control.

I request that my attending physician prescribe medication that will end my life in a humane and dignified manner.

INITIAL ONE:

_____ I have informed my family of my decision and taken their opinions into
consideration.

_____ I have decided not to inform my family of my decision.

_____ I have no family to inform of my decision.

I understand that I have the right to rescind this request at any time. I understand the full import of this request and I expect to die when I take the medication to be prescribed. I further understand that although most deaths occur within three hours, my death may take longer and my physician has counseled me about this possibility.

I make this request voluntarily and without reservation, and I accept full moral responsibility for my actions.

Signed: _____

Dated: _____

DECLARATION OF WITNESSES

We declare that the person signing this request:

(a) Is personally known to us or has provided proof of identity;

(b) Signed this request in our presence;

(c) Appears to be of sound mind and not under duress, fraud or undue influence;

(d) Is not a patient for whom either of us is attending physician.

_____Witness 1/Date

_____Witness 2/Date

NOTE: One witness shall not be a relative (by blood, marriage or adoption) of the person signing this request, shall not be entitled to any portion of the person's estate upon death and shall not own, operate or be employed at a health care facility where the person is a patient or resident. If the patient is an inpatient at a health care facility, one of the witnesses shall be an individual designated by the facility.

[1995 c.3 §6.01; 1999 c.423 §11]

PENALTIES

127.990: [Formerly part of 97.990; repealed by 1993 c.767 §29]

127.995 Penalties. (1) It shall be a Class A felony for a person without authorization of the principal to willfully alter, forge, conceal or destroy an instrument, the reinstatement or revocation of an instrument or any other evidence or document reflecting the principal's desires and interests, with the intent and effect of causing a withholding or withdrawal of life-sustaining procedures or of artificially administered nutrition and hydration which hastens the death of the principal.

(2) Except as provided in subsection (1) of this section, it shall be a Class A misdemeanor for a person without authorization of the principal to willfully alter, forge, conceal or destroy an instrument, the reinstatement or revocation of an instrument, or any other evidence or document reflecting the principal's desires and interests with the intent or effect of affecting a health care decision. [Formerly 127.585]

Glossary

aanleunwoning—independent, or assisted living section of a *bejaardenhuis* (eldercare home) or *verzorgingscentrum* (nursing home), where persons have their own apartment complete with kitchen, living room, etc. but have a call button for emergencies and residents can use the facilities of the adjacent institution, if necessary. These apartments are typically connected to a *bejaardenhuis* or *verzorginscentrum*.

Algemene Wet Bijzondere Ziektekosen (AWBZ)—General Law for Extraordinary Medical Costs. This is the law that insures each Dutch person for care and support for chronic illness, disabilities or conditions due to old age. The AWBZ covers the following seven areas: household care (cleaning, cooking and errands), personal care, nursing care, respite (to relieve family caregivers), life coaching (to help persons with disabilities live independently), rehabilitation, and residential support.

Amsterdamse Huisartsenvereniging (AHV)—Amsterdam General Practice Association

akelig—yucky, sick feeling

bejaardenhuis—home for the elderly

benauwdheid—used by patients and physicians to describe a symptom that has both physical and mental attributes. It is translated to mean "tightness of the chest," "closeness, stuffiness," "fear, anxiety," and "distress".

boodshap (*boodshappen* pl.)—shopping; errand

doel—purpose, goal, target

eenzaamheid—solitude, solitariness, loneliness; isolation, retirement, seclusion

gelukkig—happy, lucky, fortunate

huisarts (*huisartsen* pl.)—general practitioner or family doctor; literally translated to mean 'house doctor' or 'physician of the house or home'

Ik wil het niet meer—A phrase used to mean, "I don't want to [live] anymore."

Koninklijke Nederlandsche Maatschappij tot bevordering der Geneeskunst (KNMG)—the Royal Dutch Society for the Promotion of Health, formerly the Royal Dutch Medical Association

Landelijke Huisartsen Vereniging (LHV)—the National General Practice Association

lotgenoot—partner, companion (in misfortune or adversity)

Nederlandse Vereniging voor een Vrijwillig Levenseinde (NVVE)—the Dutch Association for Voluntary End-of-Life, formerly the Dutch Association for Voluntary Euthanasia

niks meer aan te doen—a phrase used typically by physician's once a patient is deemed to be terminal and their treatment phase is over. It means "there is nothing more to do or nothing more to be done."

onafhankelijk—independent

onderzoekskamer—examination room in a general practitioner's office

overleggen (overleg)—translated to mean "to consider, consult, or confer." *Overleg* is a form of group communication which aims not so much at reaching a decision as giving the parties involved the opportunity to exchange information.

prettig—pleasant, nice

slaap lekker—sleep well

spreekkamer—consultation room in a general practitioner's office *spuitje*—a syringe, refers to the injection that occurs causing a euthanasia death. Patients may say to their doctor, "*ik wil een spuitje,*" meaning they are asking for a euthanasia death.

Steun en Consultatie bij Euthanasie in Amsterdam (SCEA)—Support and Consultation for Euthanasia in Amsterdam. This is an organization of and for doctors in the greater Amsterdam area who have questions about euthanasia or need to schedule an independent, second opinion for a euthanasia or assisted suicide case.

Steun en Consultatie bij Euthanasie in Nederland (SCEN)—Support and Consultation for Euthanasia in The Netherlands. This is the national organization of and for doctors who have questions about euthanasia or need to schedule an independent, second opinion for a euthanasia or assisted suicide case.

Thuiszorg—national Dutch homecare association

verpleeghuizen—24-hour acute care nursing facility

vertrouwd—reliable, trustworthy; familiar; safe

verzorgingscentra—nursing home

References

1997. The Oregon Death with Dignity Act.

2002. Termination of Life on Request and Assisted Suicide (Review Procedures) Act. *In* Article 293, 294, 40.

2005. National Nursing Home Watch List: Accessed at http://memberofthefamily.net/usmap.htm on January 2, 2005.

AARP. n.d. What does long-term care cost? Who pays?: American Association for Retired Persons. Accessed at www.aarp.org on March 28, 2008.

AFP. 2008. Luxembourg to become third EU country to allow euthanasia: AFP. Accessed at http://afp.google.com/article/ALeqM5j_LY2E4ut3ccEXydLd0C3zlVOXFA on November 17, 2008.

Alvarez, A. 1971. The savage god: a study of suicide. New York: Bantam Books.

Anspach, Renee. 1993. Deciding who lives: fateful choices in the intensive care nursery. Berkeley: University of California Press.

AP. 2007. Frail and smiling, 'Dr. Death' walks out of prison, Vol. 2008: CNN.com http://www.cnn.com/2007/law/06/01/kevorkian.release.ap/.

Bader, Christopher D., Paul Froese, Byron Johnson, F. Carson Mencken, and Rodney Stark. 2005. The Baylor Religion Survey. Waco, TX: Baylor Institute for Studies of Religion, Baylor University.

Baer, Hans. 2001. Biomedicine and alternative healing systems in America: issues of class, race, ethnicity, and gender. Madison: University of Wisconsin Press.

Battin, Margaret P. 2005. Euthanasia and physician-assisted suicide. *In* Ending life: ethics and the way we die. M.P. Battin, ed. Pp. 17–46. New York: Oxford University Press.

———. 2008. Terminal sedation: pulling the sheet over our eyes. Hastings Center Report 38(5):27–30.

Becker, Gaylene. 1997. Disrupted lives: how people create meaning in a chaotic world. Berkeley: University of California Press.

Becker, J.W., and R. Vink. 1994. Secularisatie in Nederland, 1966–1991. 's-Gravenhage: Sociaal en Cultureel Planbureau.

Beenakker, J.J.J.M., J.C. Besteman, D.E.H. de Boer, G.J. Borger, P.A. Henderikx, H. Schoorl, C.L. Verkerk, and K. Vlierman. 1997. Holland en het water in de middeleeuwen. Hilversum: Verloren.

Behar, Ruth, and Deborah A. Gordon, eds. 1995. Women writing culture. Berkeley: University of California Press.

Binding, Karl, and Alfred Hoche. 1920. Die freigabe der vernichtung lebensunwerten lebens (The permission to destroy life unworthy of life). Leipzig: Felix Meiner Verlag.

Bourdieu, Pierre. 1992. Language and symbolic power. Cambridge: Polity Press.

Budetti, Peter P., and Teresa M. Waters. 2005. Medical malpractice law in the United States. Washington, DC: The Henry J. Kaiser Family Foundation.

CBS. 2004. One in three people in the Netherlands die in hospital: Centraal Bureau voor de Statistiek, Web Magazine. Accessed at www.cbs.nl on January 24, 2008.

———. 2007. Gezondheid en zorg in cijfers 2007. Voorburg, The Netherlands: Centraal Bureau voor de Statistiek.

———. 2008a. Old people receiving more and more care: Centraal Bureau voor de Statistiek, Web Magazine. Accessed at www.cbs.nl on January 24, 2008.

———. 2008b. Only few Dutch people go to church or mosque regularly: Centraal Bureau voor de Statistiek, Web magazine (12 June). Accessed at http://www.cbs.nl/en-GB/menu/themas/vrije-tijd-cultuur/publicaties/artikelen/archief/2008/2008-2476-wm.htm on October 23, 2008.

CC. 2005. Compassion & choices: the fight for choice at the end of life: Compassion & Choices. Accessed at http://www.compassion andchoices.org/aboutus/themovement.php on April 2, 2008.

Chabot, B.E. 2001. Sterfwerk: de dramaturgie van zelfdoding in eigen kring. Nijmegen: Uitgeverij SUN.

_____. 2007. Auto-euthanasie: verborgen stervenswegen in gesprek met naasten. Amsterdam: Uitgerverij Bert Bakker.

CIA. 2003. The world factbook: Netherlands: Central Intelligence Agency. Accessed at https://www.cia.gov/library/publications/ the-world-factbook/geos/nl.html on January 15, 2004.

Clifford, James, and George E. Marcus. 1986. Writing culture : the poetics and politics of ethnography. Berkeley: University of California Press.

CMS. 2008. Money follows the person grants: Centers for Medicare & Medicaid Services. Accessed at http://www.cms.hhs.gov/ DeficitReductionAct/20_MFP.asp on November 17, 2008.

_____. n.d. Key milestones in CMS programs: Centers for Medicare and Medicaid Services. Accessed at http://www.cms.hhs.gov/ history/dowloads/CMSProgramKeyMilestones.pdf on March 28, 2008.

CNN. 1998. Kevorkian furthers controversy with TV euthanasia tape: CNN (November 22). Accessed at http://www.cnn.com/ US/9811/22/kevorkian/index.html on October 16, 2008.

_____. 2007. Clinton unveils mandatory health care insurance plan: Cable News Network (September 18). Accessed at http://www.cnn.com/2007/POLITICS/09/17/health.care/index.ht ml on March 26, 2008.

Covinsky, KE, et al. 1994. The impact of serious illness on patients' families. JAMA 272:1939–44.

Cronon, William, ed. 1996. Uncommon ground: rethinking the human place in nature. New York: W. W. Norton & Company.

Davenport, Beverly Ann. 2000. Witnessing and the medical gaze: how medical students learn to see at a clinic for the homeless. Medical Anthropology Quarterly 14(3):310–327.

Diamond, Timothy. 1992. Making gray gold: narratives of nursing home care. Chicago: The University of Chicago Press.

DHS. 2008. Summary of Oregon's Death with Dignity Act—2007: Oregon Department of Human Services, Office of Disease Prevention and Epidemiology. Accessed at http:/oregon.gov/DHS/ph/pas/ar-index.shtml on October 16, 2008.

Dossey, Larry. 1993. Healing words. San Francisco: HarperSanFrancisco.

Douglas, Mary. 1966. Purity and danger: an analysis of concepts of pollution and taboo. London,: Routledge & K. Paul.

Dowbiggin, Ian. 2005. Euthanasia: a concise history of life, death, God, and medicine. Lanham, MD: Rowman & Littlefield Publishers, Inc.

Dunsmuir, Mollie, and Marlisa Tiedemann. 2007. Euthanasia and assisted suicide: international experience: Library of Parliament, Law and Government Division. Accessed at www.parl.gc.ca/information/library/PRBpubs/prb0703-e.htm on March 26, 2008.

Durkheim, Emile. 1912. The elementary forms of religious life. K.E. Fields, transl. New York: Free Press.

_____. 1951. Suicide, a study in sociology. Glencoe, Ill.,: Free Press.

EBS. 2005. Social values, science and technology. *In* Special Eurobarometer, Vol. 225: Directorate General Research, European Commission.

Emanuel, Ezekiel J. 1994. The history of euthanasia debates in the United States and Britain. Annals of Internal Medicine 121(10):793–802.

Emanuel, Ezekiel J., Diane Fairclough, Brian C. Clarridge, Diane Blum, Eduardo Bruera, W. Charles Penley, Lowell E. Schnipper, and Robert J. Mayer. 2000. Attitudes and practices of U.S. oncologists regarding euthanasia and physician-assisted suicide. Annals of Internal Medicine 133(7):527–532.

Faubion, James D. 1993. Modern Greek Lessons: a primer in historical constructivism. Princeton: Princeton University Press.

Firebaugh, Glenn, and Brian Harley. 1991. Trends in U.S. church attendance: secularlization and revival, or merely lifecycle effects? Journal for the Scientific Study of Religion 30(4):487–500.

Foley, Kathleen, and Herbert Hendin, eds. 2002. The case against assisted suicide: for the right to end-of-life care. Baltimore, MD: Johns Hopkins University Press.

Foucault, Michel. 1972. The archaeology of knowledge. A.M.S. Smith, transl. New York,: Pantheon Books.

———. 1978. The history of sexuality. New York: Pantheon Books.

———. 1991. The Foucault effect: studies in governmentality with two lectures by and an interview with Michel Foucault. G. Burchell, P. Miller, and C. Gordon, eds. Pp. x, 307. Chicago: University of Chicago Press.

Franklin, Sarah, and Margaret Lock, eds. 2003. Remaking life & death: toward an anthropology of the biosciences. Santa Fe: School of American Research Press.

Ganzini, Linda. 2004. The Oregon experience. *In* Physician-Assisted dying: the case for palliative care & patient choice. T.E. Quill and M.P. Battin, eds. Pp. 165–183. Baltimore: The Johns Hopkins University Press.

GAO. 2005. Social Security reform: answers to key questions. Washington, DC: U.S. Government Accountability Office, GAO-05-193SP (May).

Garsten, Ed and Reuters. 1999. Kevorkian gets 10 to 25 years in prison. *In* CNN. Pontiac, MI.

Gass, Thomas Edward. 2004. Nobody's home: candid reflections of a nursing home aide. Ithica, NY: Cornell University Press.

Gaustad, Edwin Scott. 1990. A religious history of America. San Francisco: HarperSanFrancisco.

Gennep, Arnold van. 1908. The rites of passage. [Chicago]: University of Chicago Press.

Gillick, Muriel R. 2004. Terminal sedation: an acceptable exit strategy? Annals of Internal Medicine 141(3):236–7.

Glaser, Barney G., and Anselm L. Strauss. 1965. Awareness of dying. Chicago,: Aldine Pub. Co.

———. 1968. Time for dying. Chicago: Aldine.

Gleckman, Howard. 2009. Caring for our patients: inspiring stories of families seeking new solutions to America's most urgent health crisis. New York: St. Martin's Press.

Glick, L, R. Weiss, and C.M. Parkes. 1974. The first years of bereavement. New York: Wiley.

Goffman, Erving. 1961. Asylums; essays on the social situation of mental patients and other inmates. Garden City, N.Y.,: Anchor Books.

Goldstein, Jacob. 2008. Washington passes Initiative 1000, legalizing physician-assisted suicide: Wall Street Journal Blogs (November 5). Accessed at http://blogs.wsj.com/health/2008/11/05/washington-passes-initiative-1000-legalizing-physician-assisted-suicide/ on November 5, 2008.

Gorer, Geoffrey. 1965. Death, grief, and mourning. Garden City, N.Y.: Doubleday.

Greenhouse, Linda. 2006. Supreme Court removes obstacle to assisted-suicide laws: New York Times (January 17). Accessed at http://www.nytimes.com/2006/01/17/politics/politicsspecial1/18sc otuscnd.html on October 16, 2008.

Griffin, Drew, and Kathleen Johnston. 2006. 'They pretended they were God': doctor, 2 nurses allegedly killed patients with lethal drug dose: CNN (July 19). Accessed at www.cnn.com on April 4, 2007.

Griffiths, John, Alex Bood, and Heleen Weyers. 1998. Euthanasia and law in the Netherlands. Amsterdam: Amsterdam University Press.

Griffiths, John, Heleen Weyers, and Maurice Adams. 2008. Euthanasia and law in Europe. Oxford: Hart Publishing.

Groenewegen, Peter P., and Diana M.J. Delnoij. 1997. Wat zou Nederland zijn zonder de huisarts?: Elsevier/De Tijdstroom.

Grol, Richard. 2006. Quality development in health care in the Netherlands. Nijmegen: Centre for Quality of Care Research, Radboud University Nijmegen Medical Centre.

Habermas, J. 1992. Moral consciousness and communicative action. London: MIT Press.

_____. 1996. Between facts and norms: contributions to a discourse theory of law and democracy. Cambridge: Polity Press.

Hannay, M., and M.H.M. Schrama. 1996. Van Dale handwoordenboek, Nederlands-Engels. Utrecht/Antwerpen: Van Dale Lexicografie.

Hannerz, Ulf. 2000. Thinking about culture in cities. *In* Understanding Amsterdam: essays on economic vitality, city life and urban form. L. Deben, W. Heinemeijer, and D.v.d. Vaart, eds. Pp. 161–178. Amsterdam: Het Spinhuis.

Haraway, Donna Jeanne. 2004. Crystals, fabrics, and fields: metaphors that shape embryos. Berkeley: North Atlantic Books.

Harding, Susan. 2000. The book of Jerry Falwell. Princeton: Princeton University Press.

Harrington, Charlene, Helen Carillo, Valerie Wellin, Fannie Norwood, and Nancy Miller. 2001. Access of target groups to 1915(c) Medicaid Home and Community Based Waiver Services. Home Health Care Services Quarterly 20(2):61–80.

Hasselkus, Betty Risteen. 1994. From hospital to home: family-professional relationships in geriatric rehabilitation. *In* Cultural Diversity and Geriatric Care: Challenges to the Health Professions. D.W.e. al., ed. Pp. 91–100: The Haworth Press.

Have, H.A.M.J. ten, and J.V.M. Welie. 2005. Death and medical power: an ethical analysis of Dutch euthanasia practice. Maidenhead, UK: Open University Press.

He, Wan, Manisha Sengupta, Victoria A. Velkoff, and Kimberly A. DeBarros. 2005. 65+ in the United States: 2005. Washington, DC: U.S. Census Bureau, Current Population Reports, P23–209.

Heide, A. van der, L. Deliens, K. Faisst, T. Nilstun, M. Norup, E. Paci, G. van der Wal, and P.J. van der Maas. 2003. End-of-life decision-making in six European countries: descriptive study. The Lancet 362(9381):345–350.

Heide, Agnes van der, et al. 2007. End-of-life practices in the Netherlands under the Euthanasia Act. The New England Journal of Medicine 356(19):1957–65.

Hendin, Herbert. 1997. Seduced by death: doctors, patients and assisted suicide. New York: W.W. Norton and Company.

———. 2002. The Dutch Experience. *In* The case against assisted suicide: for the right to end-of-life care. M.D. Kathleen Foley and M.D. Herbert Hendin, eds. Pp. 97–121. Baltimore: The Johns Hopkins Press.

Hingstman, L. 1999. Cijfers uit de registratie van huisartsen. Volume November. Utrecht: NIVEL.

Horst, Han van der. 2001. The low sky: understanding the Dutch. Schiedam: Scriptum Publishers.

Humphry, Derek. 1978. Jean's way. New York: Harper & Row.

_____. 1991 Final exit: the practicalities of self-deliverance and assisted suicide for the dying. New York: Dell Publishing.

_____. 2005. Farewell to Hemlock: killed by its name: Euthanasia Research & Guidance Organization (February 21). Accessed at http://www.assistedsuicide.org/farewell-to-hemlock.html on April 2, 2008.

IOM. 1997. Approaching death: improving care at the end of life. Washington, DC: National Academy Press.

ITF. 2007. Failed attempts to legalize euthanasia/assisted suicide in the United States: International Task Force on Euthanasia & Assisted Suicide. Accessed at http://www.internationaltask force.org/usa.htm on April 1, 2008.

Jalsevac, John. 2007. No charges for Hurricane Katrina doctor accused of murdering patients: LifeSiteNews (July 25). Accessed at www.lifesitenews.com/ldn/2007/jul/07072505.html on October 16, 2008.

Kaufman, Sharon. 1998. Intensive care, old age, and the problem of death in America. The Gerontologist 38(6):715–725.

_____. 2002. A commentary: hospital experience and meaning at the end of life. The Gerontologist 42(Special Issue III):34–39.

_____. 2005. … And a time to die: how American hospitals shape the end of life. New York: Scribner.

Keizer, Bert. 1996. Dancing with Mister D: notes on life and death. London: Doubleday.

Kennedy, James. 2002. Een wel-overwogen dood: euthanasie in Nederland. Amsterdam: Bert Bakker.

_____. 1995. Nieuw Babylon in aanbouw: Nederland in de jaren zestig. Amsterdam: Boom.

Keown, John, ed. 1995. Euthanasia examined; ethical, clinical and legal perspectives. Cambridge: Cambridge University Press.

Kershaw, Ian. 2001. Hitler: 1936–1945: Nemesis: W.W. Norton & Company.

Kimsma, Gerrit K., and Evert van Leeuwen. 2007. The role of family in euthanasia decision making. HEC Forum 19(4):365–373.

Kleinman, Arthur. 1980a. Patients and healers in the context of culture. Berkeley: University of California Press.

_____. 1980b. Patients and healers in the context of culture : an exploration of the borderland between anthropology, medicine, and psychiatry. Berkeley: University of California Press.

Klijn, Albert, Margaret Otlowski, and Margo Trappenburg, eds. 2001. Regulating physician-negotiated death. 's-Gravenhage: Elsevier.

Knippenberg, H. 1998. Secularization in the Netherlands in its historical and geographical dimensions. GeoJournal 45(3):209–220.

Koenig, Harold G., and Douglas M. Lawson. 2004. Faith in the future: healthcare, aging, and the role of religion. Philadelphia: Templeton Foundation Press.

Kübler-Ross, Elisabeth. 1969. On death and dying. [New York]: Macmillan.

Kuhse, H. 1992. Voluntary euthanasia in the Netherlands and slippery slopes. Bioetics News 11:1–7.

Laclau, E., and C. Mouffe. 1985. Hegemony and socialist strategy. London: Verso.

Lam, Hans. 1997. Helpen bij sterven: 'Euthanasie' in verschillende samenlevingen. Amsterdam/Overveen: Boom/Belvédère.

Langley, Alison. 2003. 'Suicide tourists' go to the Swiss for help in dying. In NYTimes.com. New York.

Lavi, Shai J. 2005. The modern art of dying: a history of euthanasia in the United States. Princeton, NJ: Princeton University Press.

Lechner, Frank J. 2008. The Netherlands: globalization and national identity. New York: Routledge.

Leman, Richard, and David Hopkins. 2004. Sixth annual report on Oregon's Death with Dignity Act. Portland, OR: Oregon Department of Human Services, Office of Disease Prevention

and Epidemiology (March 10). Accessed at www.oregon.gov/
DHS/ph/pas/ on October 16, 2008.

Leman, Richard, David Hopkins, and Melvin A. Kohn. 2006. Eighth
annual report on Oregon's Death with Dignity Act. Portland,
OR: Department of Human Services, Office of Disease Prevention and Epidemiology (March 9). Accessed at
www.oregon.gov/DHS/ph/pas/ on April 8, 2007.

Lifton, Robert Jay. 1986. The Nazi doctors: medical killing and the
psychology of genocide. NY: BasicBooks.

Lock, Margaret, and Deborah Gordon, eds. 1988. Biomedicine examined. Dordrecht: Kluwer Academic Publishers.

Lock, Margaret M. 2002. Twice dead : organ transplants and the rein-
vention of death. Berkeley: University of California Press.

Lynn, Joanne. 2004. Sick to death and not going to take it anymore! Reforming health care for the last years of life. Berkeley: University of California Press.

Maas, P.J. van der, G. van der Wal, I. Haverkate, C.L.M. de Graaff,
J.G.C. Kester, B. D. Onwuteaka-Philipsen, A. van der Heide,
J.M. Bosma, and D.L. Willems. 1996. Euthanasia, physician-
assisted suicide, and other medical practices involving the end
of life in the Netherlands, 1990–1995. The New England Journal of Medicine November 28(335):1699–1705.

Magnusson, R.S. 2004. Euthanasia: above ground, below ground.
Journal of Medical Ethics 30:441–446.

Mak, Geert. 2000. Amsterdam. P. Blom, transl. Cambridge: Har-
vard University Press.

Mamo, Laura. 1999. Death and dying: confluences of emotion and
awareness. Sociology of Health and Illness 21(1):13–36.

Meier, Diane E., Carol-Ann Emmons, Sylvan Wallenstein, Timothy Quill, R. Sean Morrison, and Christine K. Cassel. 1998. A
national survey of physician-assisted suicide and euthanasia in
the United States. The New England Journal of Medicine
338:1193–1201.

Meijer, H. n.d. Compact geography of the Netherlands. Den Bosch:
Ministry of Foreign Affairs and the Information and Documentation Centre for the Geography of the Netherlands (IDG).

Merelman, Richard M. 1984. Making something of ourselves: on culture and politics in the United States. Berkeley: University of California Press.

_____. 1991. Partial visions: culture and politics in Britain, Canada, and the United States. Madison: University of Wisconsin Press.

Minois, Georges. 1999. History of suicide: voluntary death in western culture. L.G. Cochrane, transl. Baltimore: Johns Hopkins University Press.

Morita, Tatsuya, Tatsuo Akechi, Yuriko Sugawara, Satoshi Chihara, and Yosuke Uchitomi. 2002. Practices and attitudes of Japanese oncologists and palliative care physicians concerning terminal sedation: a nationwide survey. Journal of Clinical Oncology 20(3 (February)):758–764.

Muijsenbergh, Maria Edith Teresa Catharina van den. 2001. Palliatieve zorg door de huisarts: ervaringen van huisartsen, patiënten en naastaanden, Universiteit Leiden.

NCHS. 2004. Nursing homes, beds, occupancy, and residents, according to geographic division and state: United States, 1995–2002: National Center for Health Statistics. Accessed at www.ncbi.nlm.nih.gov on April 4, 2008.

NCSL. 2008. The State of Oregon v. John Ashcroft, United States Attorney General: National Conference of State Legislatures. Accessed at www.ncsl.org/statefed/health/ORvAsh.html on October 16, 2008.

NDY. n.d. News and commentary: Not Dead Yet. Accessed at www.notdeadyet.com on April 4, 2008.

NHPCO. 2007. NHPCO facts and figures: hospice care in America: National Hospice and Palliative Care Organization (November). Accessed at www.nhpco.org/research on April 4, 2008.

Nijman, Jan. 2000. The global moment in urban evolution: a comparison of Amsterdam and Miami. In Understanding Amsterdam: essays on economic vitality, city life and urban form. L. Deben, W. Heinemeijer, and D.v.d. Vaart, eds. Pp. 19–57. Amsterdam: Het Spinhuis.

NNDB. 2008. Terri Schiavo: NNDB, Soylent Communications. Accessed at http://www.nndb.com/people/435/000026357/ on March 28, 2008.

Norwood, Frances. 1996. Disabilities and cultural diversity: a double minority identity. Society for Applied Anthropology, Atlanta, GA, 1996.

_____. 2001a. Euthanasia discourse: the changing role of the euthanasia discussion between patients and general practitioners in the Netherlands. Paper delivered at the University of Amsterdam, Social Sciences and Health Issues (SISWO) symposium, Amsterdam, The Netherlands, 2001a.

_____. 2001b. Scheduling death: euthanasia and end-of-life care in the Netherlands. Paper delivered at the Free University, Department of Social Medicine symposium, Amsterdam, The Netherlands, 2001b.

_____. 2001c. Scheduling death: the role of family and home in euthanasia and end-of-life care in the Netherlands. Paper delivered at the Annual American Anthropological Association conference (November), Washington, DC, 2001c.

_____. 2005. Euthanasia talk: euthanasia discourse, general practice and end-of-life care in the Netherlands, University of California-San Francisco and Berkeley, dissertation.

_____. 2006a. The ambivalent chaplain: negotiating structural and ideological difference on the margins of modern-day hospital medicine. Medical Anthropology 25:1–29.

_____. 2006b. A hero and a criminal: Dutch huisartsen and the making of good death through euthanasia talk in the Netherlands. Medische Antropologie 18(2):329–347.

_____. 2006c. A window into death: transforming personhood and social space through euthansia discourse and end-of-life practice in the Netherlands. Paper delivered at the Annual American Anthropological Association conference (November), San Jose, CA, 2006c.

_____. 2007. Nothing more to do: euthanasia, general practice, and end-of-life discourse in the Netherlands. Medical Anthropology 26:139–175.

NRLC. n.d. Mission statement: National Right to Life Committee. Accessed at www.nrlc.org on April 4, 2008.

NVVE. 2000. Overzicht euthanasiewetgeving. Amsterdam: NVVE.

_____. 2004. Homepage: Nederlandse Vereniging voor een Vrijwillig Levenseinde. Accessed at www.nvve.nl on October 16, 2008.

NYT. 2001. U.S. acts to stop assisted suicides: Ashcroft order is aimed at law approved by Oregon voters. *In* New York Times. Pp. A1. New York.

_____. 2005. A nation gripped by a drama of life and death. *In* New York Times. Pp. 22, column 6, section A. New York.

Obama, Barack, and Joe Biden. 2007. Barack Obama and Joe Biden's plan to lower healthcare costs and ensure affordable, accessible health coverage for all: Accessed at www.barackobama.com on October 7, 2008.

OECD. 2006. Organisation for Economic Co-operation and Development health data 2006, from the OECD Internet subscription database updated October 10, 2006. Accessed at http://www.oecd.org/health/healthdata on August 29, 2008.

Okie, Susan. 2002. 'I should die the way I want to': Oregon doctors, patients defend threatened assisted suicide law. *In* Washington Post. Pp. A1. Washington, DC.

Onwuteaka-Philipsen, B. D., et al. 2007. Evaluatie: Wet toetsing levensbeëindiging op verzoek en hulp bij zelfdoding [Evaluation of the Termination of Life on Request and Assisted Suicide (Review Procedure) Act of 2002]. The Hague: ZonMw.

Onwuteaka-Philipsen, B. D., and G. van der Wal. 1998. Steun en consultatie bij euthanasie in Amsterdam. Amsterdam: Instituut voor Extramural Geneeskundig Onderzoek/Afdeling Sociale Geneeskunde, Vrije Universiteit.

Ost, Suzanne. 2003. An analytical study of the legal, moral and ethnical aspects of the living phenomenon of euthanasia. Lewiston: E. Mellen Press.

Palriwala, Rajni. 2000. The impact of a changing social welfare system on relationship within marriage, family and social networks in the Netherlands and the public debate on this process:

Accessed at http://iias.leidenuniv.nl/iias/research/fellows/palri
wala.html on June 24, 2005.

_____. 2001. Citizenship, care, gender: renegotiations of the public and the private in the Netherlands. Leiden: Indo-Dutch Programme on Altrnatives in Development.

Pandya, Sheel. 2001. Nursing homes: fact sheet, Vol. 12/14/2007: AARP Public Policy Institute.

Paras, Eric. 2006. Foucault 2.0: beyond power and knowledge. New York: Other Press.

Parkes, Colin Murray. 1972 [1986]. Bereavement: studies of grief in adult life. Harmondsworth: Penguin.

Pearlman, Robert A., and Helene Starks. 2004. Why do people seek physician-assisted death? *In* Physician-assisted dying: the case for palliative care & patient choice. T.E. Quill and M.P. Battin, eds. Pp. 91–101. Baltimore: The Johns Hopkins University Press.

PFL. n.d. Homepage: Priests for Life. Accessed at http://www.priests forlife.org on April 4, 2008.

Pijnenborg, Loes, and PJ van der Maas. 1993. Life-terminating acts without explicit request of patient. Lancet 341(8854):1196–99.

Pool, Robert. 1996. Vragen om te sterven: euthanasie in een nederlandse ziekenhuis. Rotterdam: WYT Uitgeefgroep.

_____. 2000. Negotiating a good death: euthanasia in the Netherlands. New York: The Haworth Press.

Puchalski, Christina M. 2006. A time for listening and caring: spirituality and the care of the chronically ill and dying. Oxford: Oxford University Press.

Quill, Timothy E., and Margaret P. Battin, eds. 2004. Physician-assisted dying: the case for palliative care and patient choice. Baltimore, MD: Johns Hopkins University Press.

Ribbe, Miel W. 2004. Nursing homes in 10 nations: a comparison between countries and settings—continuing and rehabilitative care for elderly people: a comparison of countries and settings: Accessed at www.bnet.com on December 14, 2007.

Rietjens, Judith A.C., Agnes van der Heide, Astrid M. Vrakking, Bregje D. Onwuteaka-Philipsen, Paul J. van der Maas, and Gerrit van der Wal. 2004. Physician reports of terminal sedation without hydration or nutrition for patients nearing death in the Netherlands. Annals of Internal Medicine 141(3):178–185.

Rollin, Betty. 1987. Last wish: Warner.

Rutenfrans, Chris. 1997. Alles onder controle: Eerst het water, nu de dood. De Gids 7(8):576–586.

Rybczynski, Witold. 1986. Home: a short history of an idea. New York: Penguin Books.

SAL. 2001. The Sunrise story: lessons learned, lives touched, and love shared. McLean, VA: Sunrise Assisted Living, Inc.

Sankar, Andrea. 1988. Patients, physicians and context: medical care in the home. *In* Biomedicine examined. M. Lock and D.R. Gordon, eds. Pp. 155–178. Dordrecht, The Netherlands: Kluwer Academic Press.

SCBI. 2002. Euthanasia and physician-assisted suicide: recent developments and ethical analysis: Southern Cross Bioethics Institute.

Schama, Simon. 1987. The embarrassment of riches: an interpretation of Dutch culture in the golden age. New York: Vintage Books.

Scheff, Thomas. 1990. Micro sociology, discourse, emotion and social structure. Chicago: University of Chicago Press.

Scherer, Jennifer M., and Rita James Simon. 1999. Euthanasia and the right to die : a comparative view. Lanham: Rowman & Littlefield Publishers.

SCP. 2001. The Netherlands in perspective: social and cultural report 2000. The Hague: Social and Cultural Planning Office, Ministry of Health, Welfare, and Sport.

Seale, Clive. 1998. Constructing death: the sociology of dying and bereavement. Cambridge ; New York: Cambridge University Press.

SFC. 2001. Dutch way of death. *In* San Francisco Chronicle. Pp. A22. San Francisco.

Shavelson, Lonny. 1995. A chosen death: the dying confront assisted suicide. New York: Simon & Schuster.

Sheldon, Tony. 2004. Huibert Drion. British Medical Journal 328(7449):1204.

Shetter, William Z. 1987. The Netherlands in perspective: the organizations of society and environment. Leiden: Martinus Nijhoff.

Smith, Wesley J. 2001. License to kill. *In* San Francisco Chronicle. San Francisco.

Sprung, C.L., et al. 2006. Attitudes of European physicians, nurses, patients, and families regarding end-of-life decisions: the ETHICATT study. Intensive Care Medicine.

SSL. 2003. Sunrise history: Sunrise Senior Living, Inc. Accessed at http://www.sunriseseniorliving.com/about/SunriseHistory.do on September 19, 2008.

Starr, Paul. 1982. The social transformation of American medicine: the rise of a sovereign profession and the making of a vast industry. New York: Basic Books.

———. 1995. What happened to health care reform? The American Prospect 20(Winter):20–31.

Stewart, Pamela J., and Andrew Strathern. 2003. The ultimate protest statement: suicide as a means of defining self-worth among the Duna of the Southern Highlands of Papua New Guinea. Journal of Ritual Studies 17(1):79–88.

Strathern, Marilyn. 1992. After nature. Cambridge: Cambridge University Press.

Sudnow, David. 1967. Passing on; the social organization of dying. Englewood Cliffs, N.J.: Prentice-Hall.

Tännsjö, Torbjörn, ed.2004. Terminal sedation: euthanasia in disguise? Dordrecht: Kluwer Academic Publishers.

The, Anne-Mei. 1997. 'Vanavond om 8 uur …': verpleegkundige dilemma's bij euthanasie en andere beslissingen rond het levenseinde. Houten/Diegem: Bohn Stafleu van Loghum.

Thomasma, David C., and Glenn C. Graber. 1990. Euthanasia: toward an ethical social policy. New York: Continuum.

Thorpe, Kenneth E. 2004. The medical malpractice 'crisis': recent trends and the impact of state tort reforms: Health Affairs. Accessed at http://content.healthaffairs.org/cgi/content/full/hlthaff.w4.20v1/DC1 on May 27, 2008.

Turner, Victor Witter. 1967. The forest of symbols; aspects of Ndembu ritual. Ithaca, N.Y.,: Cornell University Press.

USCB. 2006. Income climbs, poverty stabilizes, uninsured rate increases. Washington, DC: U.S. Census Bureau, Public Information Office.

Vera, Hernan. 1989. On Dutch windows. Qualitative Sociology 12(2):215–34.

Verhagen, Eduard, and Pieter J.J. Sauer. 2005. The Groningen Protocol—euthanasia in severely ill newborns. The New England Journal of Medicine 352(10):959–62.

Vladeck, Bruce V. 2003. Universal health insurance in the United States: reflections on the past, present, and the future. American Journal of Public Health 93(1):16–19.

Vries, André de. 1998. Live and work in Belgium, the Netherlands and Luxembourg. Oxford: Vacation Work.

VWS. 2005. Homepage: Ministerie van Volksgezondheid, Welzijn en Sport. Accessed at www.minvws.nl on June 20, 2005.

Wal, Gerrit van der, Agnes van der Heide, Bregje D. Onwuteaka-Philipsen, and Paul J. van der Maas. 2003. Medische besluitvorming aan het einde van het leven: De praktijk en de toetsingsprocedure euthanasie. Utrecht: de Tijdstroom.

Ward, B.J., and P.A. Tate. 1994. Attitudes among NHS doctors to requests for euthanasia. British Medical Journal (May 21)(308):1332–34.

Weel, Chris van. 2004. How general practice is funded in The Netherlands. The Medical Journal of Australia 181(2):110–111.

Weyers, Heleen. 2006. Explaining the emergence of euthanasia law in the Netherlands: how the sociology of law can help the sociology of bioethics. Sociology of Health and Illness 28(6):802–816.

WHO. 2007. World health statistics: 2007. Geneva: World Health Organization.

Yanagisako, Sylvia, and Carol Delaney, eds. 1995. Naturalizing power: essays in feminist cultural analysis. New York: Routledge.

Zumthor, Paul. 1994. Daily life in Rembrandt's Holland. S.W. Taylor, transl. Stanford: Stanford University Press.

Zylicz, Zbigniew. 2002. Palliative care and euthanasia in the Netherlands: observations of a Dutch physician. *In* the case against assisted suicide: for the right to end-of-life care. K. Foley and H. Hendin, eds. Pp. 122–143. Baltimore: The Johns Hopkins University Press.

Index

abortion, xiii–xiv, 80, 81, 118
advanced directives, 84, 88, 104
AIDS
  The Netherlands, 6, 22,
    157–163, 167, 168, 176,
    180
  USA, 95, 97
Algemene Wet Bijzondere Ziektekosten [General Law for Extraordinary Medical Costs]
  (AWBZ), 14, 92, 261
Aktion T4, 80, 94
altruistic suicide
  and euthanasia, 75, 221–223
  defined, 75
Alzheimer's disease. *See* dementia
American Association for Retired Persons (AARP), 106
American Hospital Association
  (AHA), 95, 105
American Medical Association
  (AMA), 90, 104, 105
Amsterdamse Huisarstenvereniging [Amsterdam General Practice Association]

(AHV), 39
anomic suicide
  defined, 75
  and euthanasia, 75, 221–223
assisted dying, 56, 76, 231. *See also* assisted suicide, euthanasia, physician-assisted death and dying, and physician-assisted suicide
  acceptable form of suicide,
    77
  around the world, 78
  in cultural perspective,
    108–121, 226–227
  in historical perspective,
    79–108
  USA, 122
assisted suicide, 9, 10, 32, 66,
  78, 124, 148, 211, 217. *See also* assisted dying, euthanasia, physician-assisted death and dying, and physician-assisted suicide
  around the world, xvii,
    xviii, 9–10, 78
  Belgium, 9, 78

283